Atlas of
BIPOLAR DISORDERS

Dedication

This book is dedicated to the researchers and support staff, current and past, at the National Institute of Mental Health, Intramural Research Program, who are dedicated to improving the lives of people with neurobiological disorders. My years in the program provided me with mentoring, education, and professional opportunities. I will forever be grateful.

Atlas of

BIPOLAR DISORDERS

Edward H Taylor PhD LICSW

Associate Professor
School of Social Work
University of Minnesota
Twin Cities Campus, Minnesota, USA

Illustrations by

Meredith S Daniels and Carol Wiebe

School of Social Work
University of Minnesota
Twin Cities Campus, Minnesota, USA

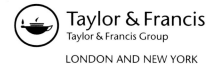
Taylor & Francis
Taylor & Francis Group

LONDON AND NEW YORK

© 2006 Taylor & Francis, an imprint of the Taylor & Francis Group

First published in the United Kingdom in 2006
by Taylor & Francis,
an imprint of the Taylor & Francis Group,
2 Park Square, Milton Park
Abingdon, Oxon OX14 4RN, UK

Tel.:   +44 (0) 20 7017 6000
Fax.:   +44 (0) 20 7017 6699
E-mail: info.medicine@tandf.co.uk
Website: http://www.tandf.co.uk/medicine

British Library Cataloguing in Publication Data

Data available on application

Library of Congress Cataloging-in-Publication Data

Data available on application

ISBN 1-84214-218-6

Distributed in North and South America by

Taylor & Francis
2000 NW Corporate Blvd
Boca Raton, FL 33431, USA

Within Continental USA
Tel.: 800 272 7737; Fax.: 800 374 3401
Outside Continental USA
Tel.: 561 994 0555; Fax.: 561 361 6018
E-mail: orders@crcpress.com

Distributed in the rest of the world by
Thomson Publishing Services
Cheriton House
North Way
Andover, Hampshire SP10 5BE, UK
Tel.: +44 (0) 1264 332424
E-mail: salesorder.tandf@thomsonpublishingservices.co.uk

Composition by Parthenon Publishing
Printed and bound by T. G. Hostench S.A., Spain

Contents

Note of Appreciation

This book was completed only because of the efforts, support, and faith of many people. I would like to give special thanks to the individuals who have worked with me throughout the project.

The following people have been friends, colleagues, and mentors for many years. They were kind enough to read and critique my proposal and chapter outlines for the book. They have been and continue to be pioneers in the study of neurobiological disorders.

Stefan Bracha, MD
Research Neuropsychiatrist,
US Department of Veterans Affairs,
National Center for Post-traumatic Stress Disorder,
Honolulu, HI, USA

Jean Cadet, MD
Branch Chief,
Molecular Neuropsychiatry Research Branch,
Intramural Research Program,
National Institute of Drug Abuse,
Baltimore, MD, USA

Frank W Putnam, MD
Professor of Pediatrics and Psychiatry,
Mayerson Center for Safe and Healthy Children,
Children's Hospital Medical Center,
University of Cincinnati,
Cincinnati, OH, USA

Numerous readings and editing of the book were done by two overworked individuals. Their insights and recommendations greatly improved the written text, and their kindness and patience are beyond my ability to express in words.

Meredith S Daniels
Coordinator,
Gamble-Skogmo Chair in Child Welfare and Youth Policy,
School of Social Work,
University of Minnesota,
Twin Cities Campus, MN, USA

Susan J Wells, PhD
Professor,
Gamble-Skogmo Land Grant Chair in Child Welfare and Youth Policy,
School of Social Work,
University of Minnesota,
Twin Cities Campus, MN, USA

Technical consultation on SPECT, computerized brain imaging, and graphic presentations was provided by the following individuals. Their guidance and expertise greatly enhanced the accuracy and depth of the book.

S Gregory Hipskind, MD, PhD
Chief Medical Officer,
Brain Matters, Inc.,
Denver, CO, USA
www.brainmattersinc.com

Michael Kelly
The Media Workshop, Inc.
1700 Lexington Avenue
Roseville, MN, USA
www.mediaworkshopmn.com

William C Klindt, MD
Founder,
Silicon Valley Brain SPECT Imaging, Inc.,
San Jose, CA, USA
www.braininspect.com

Mark Shields
Systems Administrator,
Brain Matters, Inc.,
Denver, CO, USA

Carol Wiebe
Communications Coordinator and Web Manager,
School of Social Work,
University of Minnesota,
Twin Cities Campus, MN, USA

A very special thank you goes to the family of Mine Ener. Their willingness to share this painful story, and photos, dramatically illustrates the urgent need for improving services for people and families who are unexpectedly thrust into a neuropsychiatric disorder.

Finally, I must thank the wonderful people at Taylor & Francis Medical Books. Without their help and guidance, this book would not have been possible. Producing a book requires editing, artistic skills, and business management assistance from people throughout the company. My thanks go to each of the unseen workers who have helped to pull *Atlas of Bipolar Disorders* together. A special thank you goes to Peter M Stevenson and Kelly Cornish, who have stood by my side and directed the publication process from start to finish.

Preface

Atlas of Bipolar Disorders was written to serve as a source of information for professional mental health workers, students, individuals with bipolar illness, and their families. Experienced professionals will find the book useful for reviewing current best-practice concepts, and the advancements in single photon emission computed tomography (SPECT) scanning. The treatment algorithms, medication tables, and methods for assessing undiagnosed and often hidden mania are particularly helpful for people new to the mental health professions. Neurobiological issues of this illness have been summarized, and will be helpful for social workers, psychologists, nurses, and other allied health workers who may not be overly familiar with brain studies. Chapter 4 also provides a foundation for discussing the biology of bipolar illness with patients, families, and community leaders. It is not unusual to discover that teachers, religious leaders, employers, and neighbors define the illness as a choice or psychological weakness that with effort could be overcome. Therefore, the book can provide an important service by helping people with no neuroscience training to understand that bipolar illness is a brain disorder. In a few pages, the book systematically presents easy-to-read scientific evidence illustrating that bipolar illness is not related to family, personal choices, or social environments. Furthermore, the SPECT scan images help to document that this is an illness associated with abnormalities in the brain's structure and metabolism. The book is designed to help patients and families increase their understanding of symptoms, episodes, and medications, and improve their communications with mental health professionals. Individuals and families who are aware of medication issues and

best-practice guidelines will be more educated consumers, and better able to communicate with professionals in a direct, specific, and productive manner.

In addition to offering professionals a scientific overview of bipolar disorders, the book also provides realistic clinical suggestions for planning and improving assessments and treatment interventions. Comprehensive outlines are provided for:

(1) Enhancing patient and clinician relationships;

(2) Assessing undiagnosed and hidden episodes of hypomania, and mania;

(3) Prescribing medication interventions;

(4) Assessing postpartum depression and psychosis and educating families about postpartum depression;

(5) Delivering *Systematic Eclectic Modular Therapy**.

Readers will also find two sets of questionnaires for tracking and assessing changes in symptoms and personal strengths. One set is specifically for assessing postpartum depression, and a different, but similar, set is used for monitoring bipolar symptoms.

**Systematic Eclectic Modular Therapy*© is a specific method for linking intervention modules for treating serious mental disorders. The title, *Systematic Eclectic Modular Therapy*, and the specific treatment delivery concepts and components, are copyright protected by Edward H. Taylor. Methods are outlined in this book, and detailed steps will be available in a forthcoming book.

The questionnaires may be photocopied and used without charge for patient care and research. However, they cannot be modified or published (to include electronic publications), or posted on the World Wide Web, without written permission from the author and publisher.

Whether your interest is early-onset child or adult bipolar illness, this book will provide an organized perspective of the disorders. The chapters have numerous references that will help students and other interested people to gain an in-depth knowledge of specific diagnostic, biological, and treatment issues. A combination of academic references and easy-to-read self-help books were purposely used as documentation throughout this book. Students will find the scientific references extremely helpful for writing lengthy term papers, while patients, families, and students will gain additional insights from the self-help books. For whatever reason you have picked up *Atlas of Bipolar Disorders*, it is sincerely hoped that the book will offer new insights into this complex illness, and be a constant resource for understanding treatment and patient-education issues. Finally, if one theme has to be identified for the book, it would be that scientific best-practice methods and careful diagnostic assessments cannot be accomplished without the practitioner involving, respecting, and carefully listening to the patient and each family member. Treatment of bipolar illness is best done from a team perspective that actively includes the patient and family.

Edward H Taylor
June 2005

1 Introduction and Overview

HISTORY

Throughout recorded history there have been descriptions of people with symptoms resembling bipolar illness. This is particularly true for depressive episodes. Stories depicting manic and depressive episodes can be found in ancient Greek, Persian, and biblical writings. Areteus in the second century AD recounted observing people who, for no known reason, danced throughout the night, appeared euphoric, were overly talkative and self-confident, and just as unexpectedly became sorrowful[1]. Hippocrates was well aware of depression, and insisted that what we call mental illness was caused by natural physical reasons rather than spiritual or other forces. The Greeks also identified the brain as the organ responsible for emotional disorders and intelligence. Unfortunately, by the peak of the Roman empire, scientific explanations for mental disorders gave way to mythology and religiously driven superstitions.

In the late 1600s more objective views of mental illness started gaining attention. Theophile Bonet is credited with describing patients who cycle between high and low moods. In the mid-1800s two French researchers, Falret and Baillarger, independently determined that a single form of illness could present both manic and depressive symptoms. Falret named the illness 'circular insanity', and included symptoms much as those listed in today's diagnostic manuals. He considered the illness to be genetically caused, and hypothesized that research could find a medication for relieving symptoms[1]. The work of Falret and Baillarger was built on by Emil Kraepelin. His careful systematic observations documented that mania and depression can occur in a single form of mental illness[1]. Kraepelin's 1896 textbook clinically described and named the illness manic–depressive insanity[2]. The modified term manic depression has survived through the ages, and continues to be used[1,2].

The medical progress made in the late 1800s gave way to psychoanalytical philosophy as Europe and America entered into World War II. Major disorders such as manic depression, schizophrenia, and autism were largely framed as arising from unconscious conflicts caused by parents, environments, and personal choice. Manic–depressive or bipolar symptoms were hypothesized to resolve once a patient gained insight, and chose to confront their unconscious fears, anger, and incomplete parenting[1]. The dominance of psychoanalytical talk therapy persisted in the United States for decades after World War II. This was also true throughout Europe. However, European doctors started using lithium shortly after its therapeutic properties were discovered by John F.J. Cade in the 1940s. The drug was not approved and widely available in the United States until the 1970s[1]. Today there is little debate that bipolar disorders are neurobiological diseases that are highly associated with specific and general abnormalities in the brain's structures and metabolism. A summary of brain abnormalities along with documenting single photon emission computed tomography (SPECT) scan images is presented in Chapter 4.

A COSTLY DISORDER

Bipolar disorders are a group of neurobiological disorders that historically have been associated with mild to severe shifts in mood, cognitive functions, and behaviors. Diagnostically the illness is classified throughout the industrialized world as a mood or affective disorder. A goal of this book, however, is to illustrate that bipolar disorders affect multiple neurological and body systems, creating disabilities, pain, and grief that cannot be explained in simple descriptive terms about a person's moods and emotions. This illness has biological, social, and economic repercussions. Periods of frightening manic and depressive episodes can lead to divorce, loss of job, decreased opportunities, homelessness, alcohol and substance abuse, and hardships for family members. As an example, the divorce rate among people with bipolar disorders is estimated to be 3–6 times higher than that found in the general population[3]. People suffering from bipolar disorders can only find some relief through psychiatric help and lifelong medication therapy.

The burden that a disease causes is estimated by calculating the severity of pain, suffering, disability, and deaths attributed to the disorder. In Australia the burden due to bipolar disorders was found to be greater than that associated with ovarian cancer, rheumatoid arthritis, or human immunodeficiency virus/acquired immunodeficiency syndrome (HIV/AIDS), and similar to that associated with schizophrenia[4]. The United Nations' World Health Organization (WHO) reports that bipolar illness is among the top ten causes of years lived with a disability[5]. In addition to disabilities, bipolar illness ends in suicide for many patients. Twelve percent of all suicides in Australia are committed by individuals with bipolar disorders[4], and between 10 and 15% of patients suffering with bipolar illness in the United States will take their lives[2,6]. Additional information on suicide and violence, including the dangers of postpartum depression and bipolar illness, is presented in Chapter 5.

Financially, this neurobiological disorder is estimated to cost £2 billion ($US3.8 billion) in the United Kingdom[7], $1.59 billion in Australia[4], and $45 billion in the United States annually[3]. Indirect costs account for a large proportion of the total expenditure for bipolar disorders within each of these countries. For example, in the United States, approximately $7 billion annually is spent on inpatient care and other direct costs, and $38 billion is thought to result from indirect costs such as loss of productivity[3]. Much of these costs occur because of hospitalization. However, they also represent the price of misdiagnosis, lack of community treatment, and comorbid substance abuse. The Australian study found that, on average, a correct diagnosis required 10 years from time of onset, and that patients have a 66% chance of initially receiving a wrong diagnosis[4].

Emily Dickinson

People from every walk of life have bipolar disorders. For some, mild symptom severity, or longer periods between episodes, allow reflection and creative use of their experiences. Many think that Emily Dickinson (Figure 1.1) was one of these individuals. She may have been trying to reflect on the pain of depression, and the frightening disorientation of mania, in her poems. The following verses are from *Poems of Emily Dickinson*.

I Can Wade Grief
I CAN wade grief,
Whole pools of it,
I'm used to that.

I Felt a Cleavage in My Mind
I FELT a cleavage in my mind
As if my brain had split;
I tried to match it, seam by seam,
But could not make them fit.

The thought behind I strove to join
Unto the thought before,
But sequence ravelled out of reach
Like balls upon a floor.

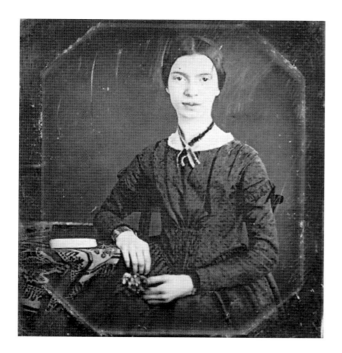

Figure 1.1   Emily Dickinson (1830–86)

A United States study found that approximately 45% of patients with bipolar illness were either untreated or improperly treated[8].

The WHO's *Project Atlas* examined worldwide mental-health resources. Using information from 185 countries, the researchers found that 41% of these countries have no mental health policy, 28% no designated mental health treatment budget, and 37% no community-care facilities. Furthermore, within countries that have a mental health policy, 57% of the plans were not initiated until the 1990s. Seventy percent of the world's population has access to less than one psychiatrist per 100 000 people. No attempt was made to estimate the accessibility for child psychiatrists[9]. The shortage of trained psychiatrists and community-care facilities predictably increases the international costs and suffering related to this disorder. Chapter 2 provides suggestions for improving diagnostic assessments. However, increasing the availability and quality of worldwide care for patients with bipolar illness and other disorders requires coordinated action by mental health professional organizations, graduate university programs, and government policy makers. Sadly, there is little motivation, or concern, within and across industrialized nations for resolving these treatment issues.

EPIDEMIOLOGY

Bipolar disorders occur worldwide. The WHO ranks bipolar disorder as the 14th highest cause of disease burden within high-income countries, and the 19th within low- and middle-income countries[10]. Prevalence estimates vary greatly within the literature. Goodwin and Jamison, reporting on epidemiology studies, found that the lifetime risk for bipolar disorder in England was 0.88%, and 1.2% for the United States[6]. The estimate for the United States, however, included both bipolar I and II. Within industrialized nations there appear to be between 9 and 15 new cases of bipolar illness per 100 000 people per year[6]. A more recent review of epidemiology studies found the lifetime prevalence rate for bipolar illness to range from a low of 0.15 per 100 persons in Hong Kong to 1.6 per 100 for both Taiwan and the United States. After controlling for numerous problems found in the epidemiological studies, the authors estimated that the worldwide prevalence for bipolar illness is approximately 0.82 per 100 people[11]. These rates, because of the strict diagnostic criteria applied, are lower than what is often seen in research and clinical publications. Unlike unipolar depression and dysthymia, bipolar I disorder is equally distributed across genders. However, rapid cycling occurs more in women than in men, and women tend to have more depressive episodes. Additionally, the onset episode in women is most often depression, while the first episode for men tends to be mania[11,12]. Men and women also differ in that, for men, manic episodes appear as much as or more often than depressive episodes[12]. Schizoaffective illness is not officially part of the bipolar disorders, but triggers mood cycles along with symptoms of schizophrenia. A person with schizoaffective disorder meets all of the diagnostic criteria for schizophrenia and a major mood disorder. There is almost no epidemiological information about this disorder. Researchers believe that it occurs in less than 1% of the general population, but may be higher in patient populations. The illness is observed more often in women than in men[12,13].

WHAT CAUSES BIPOLAR DISORDERS?

As in the case of most neurobiological illnesses, science does not have a definitive answer for this question. Perhaps more so than for any other disorder, there is mounting evidence that most individuals inherit bipolar illness. Studies of twins, family histories, and adoptions support a genetic causation hypothesis[1]. Studying identical twins has been a cornerstone for identifying genetic relationships in mental disorders. Between 1967 and 1999 there were six studies of bipolar illness in twins. Concordance rates for identical twins were reported to range from 20 to 79%, and 0 to 19% for dizygotic twin samples[14]. The study reporting 20% monozygotic concordance was methodologically flawed, and consisted of only five identical and 15 fraternal sets of twins. A concordance rate predicts the probability or odds that if one twin has bipolar disorder (or any disorder) the the other will at some point become ill. However, some researchers believe that concordance rates in the past have been inflated because of the employment of retrospective designs and overly broad diagnostic criteria. Torrey and Knable, as an example, report two recent studies with concordance rates of 43% and 44%[2]. Interpretation of the data is difficult in that one study included only seven pairs of twins. The second study with 44% concordance included 25 pairs, but has not been replicated. Nonetheless, like schizophrenia, genetics may explain causation in a large number of (but not all) cases. There may be multiple neurological pathways that lead to developing bipolar disorders. Torrey and Knable suggest that the illness, in addition to – or even in association with – genetics, may occur as a result of any of the following factors[2]:

(1) Neurological attacks from viruses, bacteria, protozoa, and fungi;

(2) Immunological factors;

(3) Neurotransmitter abnormalities;

(4) Second-messenger systems, or what is sometimes referred to as the brain's signal transduction system;

(5) Neuropeptides (endorphins, somatostatin, vasopressin, oxytocin substance P, cholecystokinin, neurotensin, and calcitonin);

(6) Body rhythm disturbances;

(7) Endocrine dysfunction.

There is varying support among scientists for these alternative explanations. The important thing for patients and family members to know is that there is no scientifically accepted evidence that families or home environments cause bipolar disorders. A detailed discussion on the role of environments and bipolar illness is provided in Chapter 2.

STRESS

Professionals, patients, and families rightfully worry about the relationship between stress and bipolar symptoms. There are numerous assumptions and hypotheses relating stress and illness onset, severity, and cycling. The research supporting any of these concepts is scanty. Stress does not appear to be a major factor in explaining why people develop bipolar disorders, nor does it relate to the number of episodes and relapses that are experienced[1,2]. There is some evidence that the first depressive or manic episode may be more influenced by stress than those that follow[1]. Nonetheless, there is little empirical support that multiple episodes are triggered by a kindling process within the brain[1,2]. Kindling refers to a dynamic interaction where the brain learns from repeated episodes to trigger future episodes automatically. This is believed to happen in seizures, but has not been documented in manic or depressive episodes. As in most physical illnesses, stress is most likely an additive interacting factor that plays a secondary role in symptom severity and quality-of-life issues.

Stress is created by perceptions, emotional responses, and internal cognitive messages or interpretations. One's perceptions are shaped not only by observations, but also by past experiences, memories, and beliefs. Bipolar illness has the ability to alter which environmental cues are influential, which memories are stimulated by events, and beliefs about observed environmental actions. Therefore, patients' perceptions of the environment vary greatly, are difficult to predict, and often are different from perceptions of others. That is, the stress experienced by a person may be more associated with and shaped by his or her bipolar illness than by current or past environmental events. Furthermore, interpreting family problems as an explanation for increased symptoms is more difficult than it appears. There is no doubt that all interpersonal relationships can be stressful, and that symptoms often increase as family arguments and problems escalate. Nevertheless, family, peer, and work relationships may have become problematic and stressed as a result of increasingly severe and unpredictable symptoms, rather than the patient's symptoms having been triggered or increased by negative environmental factors[1,2]. Additional details about stress and bipolar illness can be found in Chapter 2.

WHO SHOULD ONE SEE FOR HELP?

Bipolar illness is a complicated disease that cannot be cured. As in diabetes, for example, the symptoms must be managed, and are often controlled to the point that people live full and meaningful lives. However, because bipolar illness is lifelong, occurs in episodes, requires multiple forms of intervention, and can quickly change, it is best treated by a mental health team. Patients will find it helpful if the medical, educational, social, case management, advocacy, and psychotherapy interventions are handled by a collaborating team of experts. Nonetheless, treatment without appropriate medication is doomed. Not only will it fail, but in most cases it will result in patients experiencing increased symptoms. At a minimum, treatment requires individuals and their families to have an ongoing positive relationship with a psychiatrist who can medically respond to shifting and changing bipolar symptoms. Other parts of the treatment regimen, such as education, community support, family problem-solving sessions, and appropriate psychotherapies, can be handled by any mental health professional knowledgeable about bipolar disorders and experienced in the required treatment services. Some of the professions trained to provide diagnostic assessments, screenings, and interventions other than medication treatments include clinical social workers, psychologists, and psychiatric nurses. Specialized and highly

targeted rehabilitation assistance is often provided by occupational, recreational, movement, and vocational rehabilitation therapists. The key for treatment is locating psychiatrists and other mental health professionals who have studied and treated bipolar illness. These issues are further developed Chapter 6.

REFERENCES

1. Taylor EH. Manic-depressive illness. In Ramachandran VS, ed. Encyclopedia of the Human Brain. San Diego: Academic Press, 2002; 2: 745–57.

2. Torrey EF, Knable MB. Surviving Manic Depression: A Manual on Bipolar Disorder for Patients, Families and Providers. New York: Basic Books, 2002.

3. Dunner DL. Clinical consequences of under-recognized bipolar spectrum disorder. Bipolar Disord 2003, 5: 456–63.

4. Access Economics; SANE Australia. Bipolar Disorders: Costs: An Analysis of the Burden of Bipolar Disorder and Related Suicide in Australia. Melbourne, 2003.

5. Murray CJ, Lopez AD, eds. The Global Burden of Disease: A Comprehensive Assessment of Mortality and Disability From Diseases, Injuries, and Risk Factors in 1990 and Projected to 2020. Cambridge: Harvard University Press, 1996.

6. Goodwin FK, Jamison KR. Manic–Depressive Illness. Oxford: Oxford University Press, 1990.

7. Gupta RD, Guest JF. Annual cost of bipolar disorder to UK society. Br J Psychiatry 2002; 180: 227–33.

8. Birnbaum H, Greenberg P, Huang Z, et al. Drug treatment patterns of bipolar disorder and associated costs. In National Institute of Mental Health's 44th Annual New Clinic Drug Evaluation Unit (NCDEU). Washington, DC: NIMH, 2004: 106.

9. World Health Organization. Fact Sheet: Project Atlas: Mapping Mental Health Resources Around the World. New York: United Nations, World Health Organization, 2001: 1–4.

10. World Health Organization. Mental Health and Substance Abuse, Including Alcohol in the South-East Asia Region of WHO. New Delhi: World Health Organization, Regional Office for South-East Asia, 2001: 1–22.

11. Waraich P, Goldner EM, Somers JM. Prevalence and incidence studies of mood disorders: a systematic review of the literature. Can J Psychiatry 2004, 49: 124–38.

12. American Psychiatric Association. Diagnostic and Statistical Manual of Mental Disorders, 4th edn, Text Revision. Washington, DC: American Psychiatric Association, 2000.

13. Ho B-C, Black DW, Andreasen NC. Schizophrenia and other psychotic disorders. In Hales RE, Yudofsky SC, eds. The American Psychiatric Publishing Textbook of Clinical Psychiatry, 4th edition. Washington, DC: American Psychiatric Publishing, 2003: 379–438.

14. Jones I, Kent L, Craddock N. Genetics of affective disorders. In McGuffin P, Owen MJ, Gottesman II, eds. Psychiatric Genetics and Genomics. Oxford: Oxford University Press, 2003: 211–47.

2 Presentation and Classification of Bipolar Disorders

DEFINING THE ILLNESS

Bipolar disorder, sometimes called manic depression, is a series of related neurobiological illnesses. Popular writers and news announcers simply describe the disorder as an illness causing people to experience extreme emotional lows and at other times wild euphoric highs. As with most generalizations, this fails to communicate the true experience, pain, and cost of the illness. Brief definitions also invite people to picture a simplified problem controllable by will and choice. Bipolar disorder is easy to define, but difficult to explain in a way that effectively communicates its overwhelming destructive power. Explanations that blame demons, unconscious motives, poor parenting, or God have largely disappeared throughout industrialized nations. Yet, for many, depressive and manic symptoms are seen as behavioral choices. The idea that mental disorders can take away a person's free will continues to be difficult for people to accept intellectually and emotionally.

The culture and politics of self-reliance have led many community leaders and policy-makers to frame bipolar illness as a cognitive struggle between right and wrong. Perhaps the last dragon to be slain is in helping the public as well as patients and families to understand that bipolar illness is not a voluntary condition. It is not possible to think, exercise, or behave your way out of this illness. As with any illness, optimism, spirituality, support, and determination may improve quality of life and enhance treatment effectiveness. However, the reality is that bipolar disorders hold a person hostage, reduce introspection and problem-solving skills, and dictate cognitions, feelings, perceptions, and behaviors.

Environments are important in the treatment of a bipolar disorder, but offer little in understanding of the origins or the illness. Furthermore, assessing the contribution made by environmental settings to a person's level of severity of the illness is difficult. The nature of a bipolar disorder is to alter how patients perceive and experience their surroundings. A common understanding of psychiatric disorders, environmental factors, and life events is illustrated in Figure 2.1. The difficulty with this illustration is that emotional responses and environmental elements appear to be both separate and equal in explaining bipolar episodes and remission.

There is no question that many factors outside a person's biology interact with and influence symptoms. Nonetheless, resilience against the onset of a bipolar disorder and potential for remission are subordinate to a person's neurobiological health. The brain's physical ability to respond to medication and accept environmental support are the major factors in determining prognosis. Changes in the brain associated with a bipolar disorder alter how the world is perceived, understood, and experienced. Therefore, gaining a goodness-of-fit between people with bipolar illness and environmental settings is difficult. What appears to be supportive to the care-provider may be perceived and translated as dangerous, insulting, or rejecting by a person whose brain has been structurally and functionally altered. The power of the environment to influence symptoms is compromised by the severity of changes, insults, and overall abnormalities in the patient's brain (Figure 2.2). As a result, supportive settings, positive surroundings, and milieu may decrease, increase, or have little effect on bipolar symptoms.

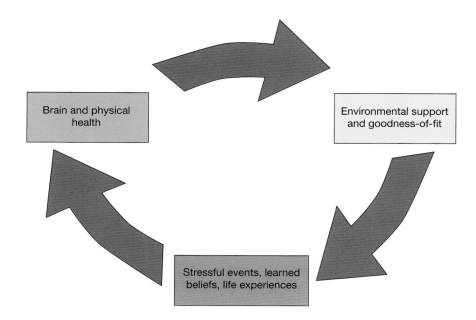

Figure 2.1 Typical interactive model for explaining symptom formation and change. While these and other factors interact and influence bipolar illness, they do not have equal power for causing or reducing symptoms

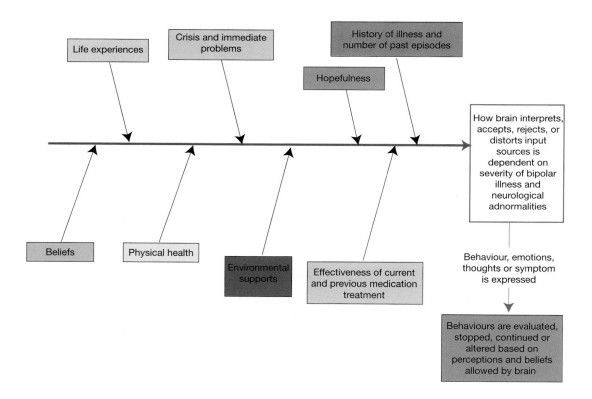

Figure 2.2 Bioecological perspective of bipolar symptoms. As the brain receives imput from numerous factors, it processes and acts on the information. The ability for each factor to interact and influence actions is dependent on the severity of the illness and brain abnormality. During episodes, both positive and negative input may be perceived differently and altered from their actual meaning and reality. When this occurs the person has almost no choice but to act on the information as processed and presented

People have difficulty in understanding bipolar illness because it resembles a chameleon. Symptoms shift within and between diagnostic subtypes. Manic or depressive symptoms can be over in a day, or last considerably longer than a month. Severity and symptoms change from episode to episode and people with identical diagnoses experience a disorder differently. Additionally, difficulties and symptoms may range from almost undetectable to so severe that the only chance for survival is hospitalization. Family members and others may also challenge the veracity of a person's symptoms as the individual's level of functioning returns to normal between episodes. Moreover, observers often do not perceive that bipolar illness attacks the person's whole being. After all, everyone has periods of sadness and moments of exuberance. The community is left without experiences and words for comprehending how bipolar disorders go beyond personal experiences such as grief, disappointment, and extreme delight. Therefore, patients are better served when bipolar illness is explained as consisting of more than emotional turmoil and degrees of sadness or excitement. More than an illness of emotions, this is a dynamic brain disorder that robs patients of their ability to identify alternative life solutions, triggers physical, cognitive, emotional, and behavioral problems, and can result in death. As shown in Figures 2.1 and 2.2, bipolar disorder can cause reductions in, among other things, physical motor coordination, information processing, abstract thinking, and technical and social skills.

BIPOLAR DISORDER SUBTYPES

The following diagnostic categories are listed by the American Psychiatric Association as forms of bipolar illness: cyclothymic, bipolar II, bipolar I, and bipolar disorder not otherwise specified (NOS)[1].

Additionally, a growing number of researchers and clinicians include schizoaffective disorder as part of the bipolar spectrum[2]. Individuals with schizoaffective disorder meet the requirements for a diagnosis of schizophrenia, and all of the criteria for having a major depressive, manic, or mixed mood episode. The *Diagnostic and Statistical Manual of Mental Disorders* (DSM-IV-TR) does not include schizoaffective disorder as a form of bipolar illness. However, a person who has an occurrence of mania or a mixed episode along with schizophrenia is classified as having schizoaffective disorder, bipolar type.

DEFINING AN EPISODE

The concept of episodes is key to understanding and diagnosing bipolar disorders. Symptoms appear in clusters and remain active over a period of time and then go into remission. Diagnosis is based upon

---

There is Hope

Bipolar disorders create many ongoing difficulties and hardships for patients and families. The illness, however, is not without hope. Individuals coping with the disorder may find it helpful periodically to remind themselves that:

- People often return to their pre-illness level of functioning after an episode ends.

- Medication significantly reduces symptoms for a majority of people with a bipolar disorder.

- Genetic mapping is opening new doors for understanding bipolar disorders.

- The neurobiological secrets of bipolar illness are being rapidly discovered by researchers.

- Increasing knowledge about bipolar disorders will bring new and improved treatment for many people within their lifetimes.

- Through many avenues the general public are learning that bipolar disorders are biological illnesses that should not be stigmatized.

- In spite of this illness, many people, as evidenced by famous people with a bipolar disorder, not only survive, but contribute to society.

documenting that a person cycles from a state of normal functioning into a period where a cluster of symptoms is observed and measured, and then returns to, or near, that person's normal baseline. In other words, an episode requires:

(1) Moving from a baseline of relatively normal functioning to a state of reduced skills or increased cognitive, emotional, or behavioral difficulties;

(2) Having a cluster of symptoms that are observable and measurable;

(3) Having a cluster of symptoms that meet established diagnostic criteria;

(4) Having symptoms and functional problems that are time-limited;

(5) Having remission of symptoms and a return to or near to the pre-episode level of functioning.

Identifying exactly when an episode starts and ends is often difficult. Nonetheless, most episodes have three parts that are known as the prodromal, active, and recovery phases[3]. In the prodromal phase symptoms range in severity from extremely mild to moderate.

The awareness of symptoms existing in the prodromal phase varies among people, but most recognize that a problem is developing as the symptoms move toward the upper limits of mild severity. However, throughout the prodromal phase patients often try to 'tough it out.' Some simply hope that the difficulties will go away or at least not increase, while others do not seek professional help out of fear. When symptoms are extremely mild, patients often worry about being labeled a complainer or about having medication, psychotherapy, or hospitalization forced on them. Early intervention, perhaps as mild as decreasing social and work obligations and starting or adding medication, may prevent the person from going into a full episode. The prodromal phase is followed by an active phase where symptoms reach their apex of severity. How long the episode remains active before moving into the final phase of recovery or remission is almost impossible to predict. Within bipolar disorders each manic, hypomanic, mixed, or depressive episode can last a matter of days or months. Once in remission, the amount of time between episodes is highly variable. Unfortunately, this is a chronic recurring illness. Without treatment a manic episode can last 3 or more months, and depression even longer[4]. Additionally, between episodes, residual symptoms cause problems in daily functioning and adjustment difficulties for over 50% of people with a bipolar disorder. Approximately 10–15% of all patients experience almost continuous severe difficulties in managing part of their daily routine and responsibilities[5]. With time and treatment most patients improve and decrease their number of episodes.

BIPOLAR I DISORDER

Bipolar I disorder is the most severe form of illness in the spectrum. It most often starts in late adolescents and young adulthood (Figure 2.3).

Bipolar I symptoms can range from extremely severe depression to equally severe mania (Figure 2.4).

Patients are diagnosed with bipolar I if they have had at least one manic or mixed episode. However, the mania cannot have been induced by medications or other somatic treatments for depression, substance abuse, toxins, or a general medical condition[1]. A number of medical conditions can cause both mania and depression, including strokes, epilepsy, infections, and medication interaction.

Mania is a psychiatric condition in which one's mood switches from normal to an almost constant

---

Depression is Coming

If a person has a documented manic episode but no depression, a diagnosis of bipolar I is nonetheless given. Statistically the individual has a high probability of experiencing a major depressive episode at some point in their life.

Additionally, patients may present with mania, but also have previously had an untreated depressive episode. This is particularly true for people who have a history of abusing alcohol and other substances. They may have unknowingly been self-medicating with alcohol and 'street' drugs.

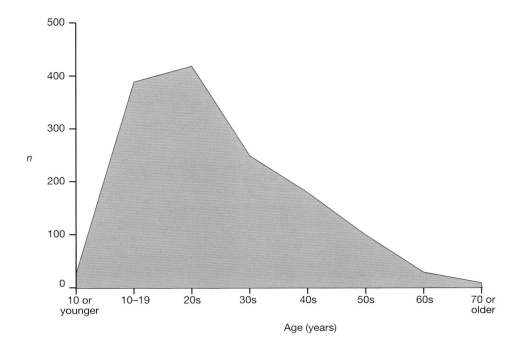

a

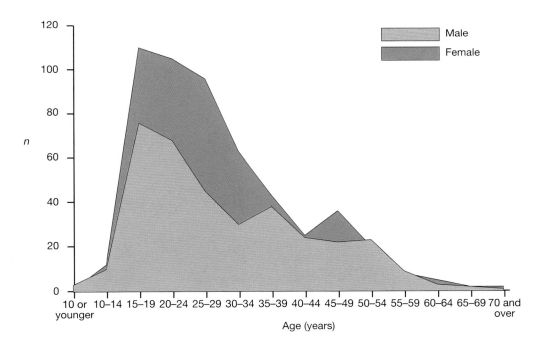

b

Figure 2.3 Bipolar disorder. (a) Age of onset. (b) Ages of onset for women and men are similar. The mean onset age according to Goodwin and Jamison is around 19, and the average age of first treatment for bipolar illness is approximately 22 years. Adapted from Figures 6.1 and 6.2 from *Manic–Depressive Illness* by Frederick K. Goodwin and Kay R. Jamison, copyright © 1990 by Oxford University Press, Inc. Used by permission of Oxford University Press, Inc.

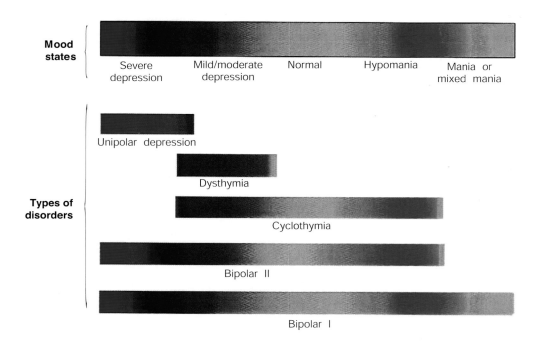

Mood states

Severe depression | Mild/moderate depression | Normal | Hypomania | Mania or mixed mania

Types of disorders

Unipolar depression

Dysthymia

Cyclothymia

Bipolar II

Bipolar I

Figure 2.4 The mood spectrum: illustrates and compares range of severity for bipolar disorders

Table 2.1 Examples of manic symptoms

Symptom	Symptom impact/effect
Energy	boundless: works fast for long hours or takes on extra tasks, does not appear to experience fatigue
Sleep	greatly decreased night after night
Self-perception	inflated, often grandiose ideas, believes knowledge or skills are greater than those of others'
Mood	euphoria to irritability; unrealistic optimism that is highly self-focused, euphoria and optimism that are out of context and do not seem to dissipate
Attention/concentration	easily distracted, focuses on unimportant details, extremely impulsive
Psychomotor activity	most often highly increased: high agitation
Goals	increased and overstated
Thinking	poor judgment, racing thoughts, often incomplete thoughts or missing steps in logic and planning
Dress	dress changed to an unusual, daring, or strange style
Speech	rapid-firing pressured speech, talking over other people's statements, not letting people complete statements, louder and more constant streams of speech, will not stop talking, jumps from topic to topic
Risk-taking behaviors	high: unusual, reckless, not characteristic of the person, confrontational and aggressive; involved in physical and verbal fights; engages in sex with multiple partners
Activity	pleasure-seeking, compulsively doing tasks such as cleaning for extended hours; gambling
Psychosis	auditory or visual hallucinations, paranoid or other delusions

state of overactive thoughts and behaviors, abnormal euphoria, or irritation for a week or more. Typical symptoms are described in Table 2.1. To meet the criteria for a formal diagnosis the mania must significantly decrease a person's social, school, or work skills. As the symptoms increase, patients are unable to complete their routine tasks.

Often, hospitalization is needed to protect the person from hurting her- or himself accidentally or on purpose. Manic symptoms can escalate extremely quickly. This is especially true when the patient has become aggressive or agitated, is participating in high-risk behaviors, or becomes psychotic. Hospitalization may be needed immediately for

The Experience of Mania

Explanation

This is an exercise that the author uses with graduate students studying psychopathology. The idea is to help people recognize bits and pieces of manic behavior that have occurred in their own private lives, and mentally combine them into a simulation of mania. Obviously a simulation cannot tell us what mania is like. One must live the experience to know and understand truly how it feels. The exercise, however, can help us to better understand the way that mania grows and takes over the mind. Most people will not relate to all of the suggested images. When an experience or image is suggested that does not match your past, simply accept that it is a factor that often occurs during a manic episode.

Exercise

Recall a time when exuberant energy caused a momentary lapse in judgment. Perhaps in excitement you embarrassingly overrated your work, claimed phantom skills, or exaggerated personal influence and relationships. Picture the time you acted silly, insulting, or hyperactive, or took physical risks that could have ended in disaster. Picture the time you took chances driving fast, weaving through traffic, accepted a dare that could have ended in death, or that time you had unprotected sex with a stranger. Perhaps after sleeping only a couple of hours for one or two nights you were over-talkative, found the unfunny comical, then suddenly became irritable, angry, and hurt over something that now makes no sense. Remember becoming verbally aggressive and making threatening remarks, perhaps shoving another person for no real reason. Finally, picture a time when, with friends, perhaps partly intoxicated, you insisted on weaving a conspiracy story. With no effort, one thought after another rushed into your head and out of your mouth. At the time every fast-moving detail seamlessly fitted together. Today, embarrassment is still felt when friends joke about the improbable logic loosely knitted into an unbelievable fantasy.

Now, imagine all of these exaggerated thoughts, emotions, and behaviors coming together at once. The flood of ideas are welcomed until sleepless nights and unstoppable thinking turn self-assurance into fear and confusion. Unfinished thoughts start rapidly colliding, crashing like freight trains, and leaving you disorientated, irritated, and unsure how to end the madness. The feelings of understanding the unknowable are suddenly gone, creating a void filled only by never-ending unfinished, unthinkable thoughts. Feel the fear and confusion washing over you when no explanation for these emotions, thoughts, and behaviors is found. Picture yourself overwhelmed with anxiety, stressed beyond any point ever experienced, when a plan for escaping, returning to normalcy and sanity will not come into your mind. You now know that thinking your way back to reality is impossible.

You feel hopelessly alone, frightened, confused, unable to stop the noise in your mind, control your emotions, thoughts, and body. You are pacing, talking faster than ever, but saying nothing, thinking thoughts that have no meaning, crying, yelling for at people for no real reason. You want to run and hide and be found all at the same time. You feel hot and cold, want to take all your clothing off yet wear everything you own. You move about having no idea where you are going. You are not sure what you want or what to do. You are terrified with no answers. You are having a manic episode.

patients who are spiraling out of control, even if their symptoms have not been present for a full week.

BIPOLAR I AND DEPRESSIVE EPISODES

Researchers have documented that at some point in a person's life after they have had a manic episode, depression will appear (Figure 2.5)[8]. However, there is evidence that a few people never cycle into depression, or are prone to having more episodes of whichever mood pole occurs at the time of onset. That is, if mania occurs first, a person has a higher probability of having more manic episodes over a lifetime than bipolar depression episodes.

The opposite is true if a patient's first episode is depression[8]. Goldberg and Kocsis reviewed the research literature and found there to be a 5–40% chance that patients who have a major depressive episode will at some point meet the criteria for bipolar disorder. The probability for a depressed person to develop manic or mixed episodes increases if the depression occurred as a child or adolescent, it occurred rapidly at onset, the illness included psychomotor retardation or other atypical depressive symptoms, or the depression was comorbid with psychosis[8]. Episodes do not have to alternate in polarity. A person may have a series of depressions or manic attacks before experiencing the opposite

mood. Therefore, predicting what type of episode will come in the future is difficult.

Depression is more than sadness. The DSM-IV-TR requires four or more major symptoms plus an observable depressed mood or loss of interest in previously pleasurable activities before a major depressive episode is diagnosed. In addition, the symptoms must have been present for at least 2 weeks, and have significantly decreased the individual's routine level of functioning[1]. Examples of typical symptoms triggered by depression are given in Table 2.2.

Like mania, depression can cause agitation and aggression. However, suicide and self-harm are more common during depressive episodes than is violence to others. In rare cases, depressed patients may purposely injure or kill another person (see Chapter 5).

MIXED EPISODE

A mixed episode (Figure 2.6) consists of symptoms, emotions, and behaviors that meet the DSM-IV-TR criteria for both major depressive and manic episodes on most days for at least 1 week. Patients may experience symptoms such as sadness, hopelessness, periods of crying, or suicidal thoughts, while simultaneously having unrealistic energy, and

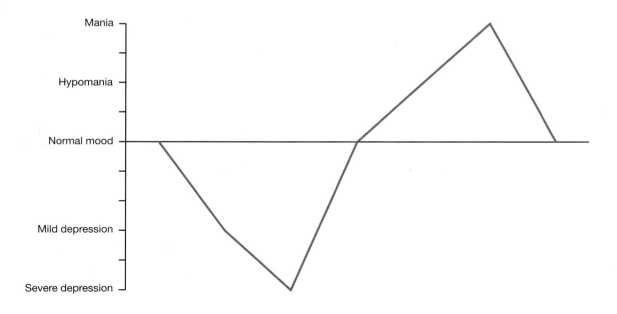

Figure 2.5 Bipolar I disorder. Adapted from reference 7

Table 2.2 Examples of depression symptoms

Symptom	Symptom impact/effect
Energy	reduced, often tired, hard to refuel
Sleep	sleep too much or cannot sleep; fall asleep and wake after a couple of hours and cannot return to sleep
Somatic problems	complaints of stomach problems, constipation, aches and pains appearing to have no relationship to medical problems
Interest and pleasure	reduced
Eating	either greatly decreased or increased food intake, overall diet often unhealthy
Psychomotor skills	greatly slowed or increased agitation
Self-perception	greatly reduced, may experience guilt or worthlessness
Cognitive skills	information processing slowed, concentration reduced, decision-making difficult, working memory decreased
Mood/emotions	sadness most of the time, anger, loss of any emotional feelings, reports of emotional pain, feeling empty, crying for no reason or inability to cry
Anxiety	elevated
Self-care and family responsibilities	hygiene may decrease; attention and responsibilities to family members decrease, children may be at risk for neglect
Hopelessness	High; high possibility of suicidal thoughts

euphoria. Either the symptoms can co-occur, lying virtually on top of each other, or patients can immediately, with no relief, cycle from one mood to another. Moods that switch, one episode after another, and neither blend together nor allow the patient to regain a completely normal state, may be ultradian cycling rather than a true mixed episode. This is a form of rapid cycling occurring over hours or days. It is not unusual for mixed states and ultradian cycling to immediately follow each other[9].

When the moods blend together, a patient may, for example, feel tired and unable to get out of bed, yet also have grandiose and racing thoughts. Mixed episodes often include agitation, insomnia, appetite changes, psychosis, and suicidal thoughts. This is a dangerous period of time because extreme feelings of depression interact with manic energy, and increase the possibility of suicide or violence to others. Additionally, this can be a terrifying time for the patient. Kay Jamison described her mixed episodes as follows[10]:

On occasion, these periods of total despair would be made even worse by terrible agitation. My mind would race from subject to subject, but instead of being filled with ... exuberance and cosmic thoughts ... it would be drenched in awful sounds and images of decay and dying; dead bodies on the beach, charred remains of animals, toe-tagged corpses in morgues.

The mixed state described by Jamison is referred to by clinicians as agitated depression. It contains a high level of energy and agitation combined with depressed or poverty of thought. Kraepelin originally called this type of symptom mixing excited depression[11]. Patients who have some manic symptoms but no euphoria, and demonstrate restlessness along with other symptoms of depression, are thought to have dysphoric mania[11]. This type of mixed state is seen mostly in women, and has been found to be an indicator of a higher probability for suicide and poorer response to lithium[9]. Currently, the professional community is debating whether diagnosing a mixed episode should require meeting all DSM-IV-TR criteria for manic and major depressive episodes. This may be overly restrictive and exclude people who have only one or two elements of each pole

The Experience of Depression*

Explanation

This is a continuation of the first exercise. This time you are asked to allow your mind to explore and sample what it is like to have a major depressive episode. You will be guided through a series of suggested feelings and mental images that simulate a clinically depressed mood. Obviously a simulation cannot tell us what real depression is like. The exercise, however, can help us better to understand how depression capture's the mind and removes choices. You are again reminded that most people do not relate to all of the suggested images. When an experience is suggested that does not match your past, simply accept that it is a factor that often occurs during a depressive episode

Exercise

We all become sad and blue, but this is not depression. To understand depression, picture day after day, week after week, finding no joy or peace in anyone or anything. Successes are either experienced as failures, or just added burdens, more obligations, piled upon an already tired body. Every movement, thought, action takes effort and seems to occur in slow, random spasms. Processing or even understanding information requires purposeful attention. Maintaining focus as others talk, or reading a few sentences, is almost impossible. Every negotiation, task, and interpersonal exchange feels like physical labor. Yet no one perceives how hard you are working, how tired you feel, how stress hangs everywhere.

You simultaneously experience a sense of heavy, anesthetizing dullness and psychic emotional pain that cannot be relieved. Only sleep ends the tormenting sensations, but remaining asleep for more than an hour or two is impossible. At other times you lie in bed either sleeping or awake, exhausted, unable to move most of the day. All the time you are in bed, thoughts about unfinished tasks and personal failures repeatedly burn in your mind. However, neither energy to move, nor a plan for prioritizing and resolving these tasks, comes to mind. There is no solution. The pain and dullness are always there, fading together into a constant radiating fire. Yet, no matter what anyone claims, you know the pain is real. Your stomach has that shocked constant feeling of being upset, and pains randomly shoot through your chest, mimicking a heart attack. Even your coordination has slowed and periodically refuses to work. As a result, things are dropped, dishes broken, written notes scribbled, nothing works like it did! Perhaps most frightening is that you feel dead inside, nothing fills the emptiness.

There is no room, no energy for discovering alternative ideas. However, frustration is quickly turning to acceptance. Therapists, doctors, family, and friends will never grasp that you are in an invisible box that cannot be penetrated. Your mind searches, but there simply is no way out of the box, it is hopeless. You are witnessing your own demise and have no means to control or change the direction being traveled. But it does not really matter. After all, you reason, one must finally accept that there are no answers, there is no escape. The tears have stopped, crying would bring relief, but both are impossible. A nagging awareness that there are no joys, no delighting colors and sounds, no wonderful smells and tastes, no answers, no future, only burden and failure, hardships, pain, and death: death to stop the pain, death because the mind demands death for reasons neither known nor understood, but nonetheless demanded and required. This is depression.

*Constructed from statements made to the author by people with bipolar disorder.

occurring simultaneously[9,11]. The argument gains importance when one considers that between 30 and 50% of all manic episodes include some depressive symptoms[9]. Furthermore, most patients with agitated depression or dysphoric mania would not qualify for the diagnosis of a mixed episode under the present requirements.

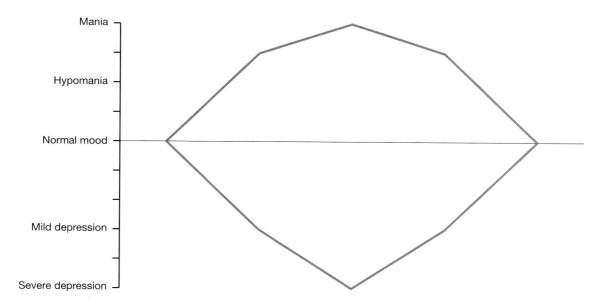

Figure 2.6 Mixed episode. Adapted from reference 7

RAPID CYCLING

Approximately 10–20% of patients with bipolar I or bipolar II develop what is known as rapid cycling. Within the group having rapid cycling episodes, 70–90% are women. This means that the person experiences four or more episodes of major depression, mania, mixed state, or hypomania as defined by DSM-IV-TR in a 12-month period[1]. Rather than mixing in a simultaneous or blended manner, the mood episodes are distinctly separate, but return one after another throughout the year. The episodes can appear in any combination or order (Figure 2.7).

As an example, a depressive episode can follow other depressive episodes. There must, however, be a period of full remission between each episode, or a switch in polarity. DSM-IV-TR identifies mania, hypomania, and mixed episodes as being clustered at the manic pole. This means that a patient who has a manic episode followed immediately by hypomania or a mixed state has had only one episode that counts toward the four needed for diagnosing rapid cycling, whereas a patient who moves from a manic episode without remission into a major depression has experienced two separate episodes[1]. This is because when two episodes immediately follow each other, and are part of the same pole or cluster of symptoms, there is a strong probability that they are actually the same episode. Rapid cycling is an indica-tor or predictor that the patient will have more severe symptoms, and not respond well to lithium and other medications traditionally used for treating bipolar illness.

BIPOLAR II DISORDER

It is a mistake to think of bipolar II as simply a milder form of bipolar I illness. Both are serious mental disorders that have the ability to disable patients and cause hardships for their families. Bipolar II disorder is diagnosed if individuals have one or more major depressive episodes, and at least one episode of hypomania (Figure 2.8). Hypomania is present when the patient has an abnormally elevated, expansive, or irritable mood for at least 4 days. The change in mood must also be accompanied by three of seven symptoms identified by DSM-IV-TR[1]. These symptoms are similar to the criteria listed for assessing a manic episode. Bipolar II disorder has a lifetime prevalence of about 0.5%[1,9]. The primary differences between mania and hypomania are that with the latter the patient remains more organized, appears less bizarre, and has less overall cognitive and affective impairment. As a result, hypomanic episodes may make a person difficult to be around, but do not substantially reduce their ability to function at work or home, and hospitalization is seldom required[1,11].

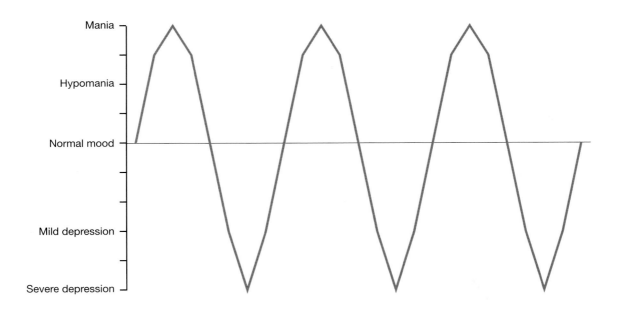

Figure 2.7 Rapid cycling (occurs within 1 year). Adapted from reference 7

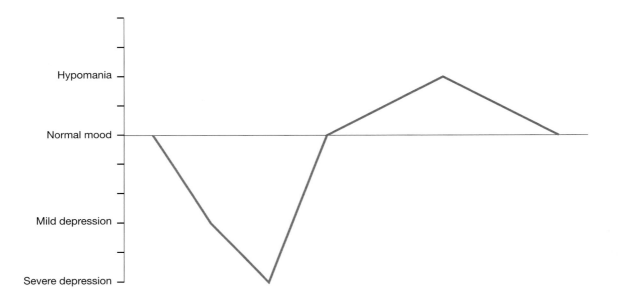

Figure 2.8 Bipolar II disorder. Adapted from reference 7

Keep in mind that this diagnosis cannot be given if the person has at any time had a manic or mixed episode. If a patient is currently in the midst of a hypomanic episode, but previously has had a manic or mixed episode, the patient would be assessed as having bipolar I. In addition to the severity of mania, bipolar I and II differ in several other ways. More females are diagnosed with bipolar II than are males, but bipolar I is about evenly distributed between men and women. Hypomanic episodes (60–70%) occur immediately before or after a major depressive episode[1]. Bipolar I patients may have long periods before experiencing both a manic and a depressive episode. Both bipolar I and II patients can develop rapid cycling, but only bipolar I patients have mixed episodes. The criteria for rapid cycling are identical for both disorders. There is also evidence that suicide is a significant risk factor during depressive episodes (see Chapter 5)[1,9]. Most people who have bipolar II will live their lives without developing a more severe form of bipolar illness. Unfortunately, within a 5-year period, approximately 5–15% of individuals with bipolar II illness will have a manic episode and meet the criteria for a diagnoses of bipolar I.

CYCLOTHYMIA

Cyclothymia is the mildest yet most persistent form of bipolar illness. It often first occurs in the teen years and early adulthood. Lifetime prevalence for the disorder is between 0.4 and 1%[1,9]. A person with cyclothymia has elements of hypomania and depression, but the symptoms never meet the criteria to be characterized as a hypomanic or major depressive episode (Figure 2.9). Cyclothymia shifts between symptoms of hypomania such as inflated self-

esteem, or irritability, and indicators of depression such as reduced energy and sleep disturbances. However, the symptoms fail to meet the requirements to be classified as full-blown episodes. This may occur because there are not enough symptoms, or the problems lack severity or do not last long enough to meet time requirements[1].

While the symptoms are milder than in other forms of bipolar disorder they almost never leave the person. Cyclothymia becomes a way of life. A major part of the diagnostic criteria is that in a 2-year period the patient cannot have a symptom-free interval lasting more than 2 months[1]. Additionally, during the initial 2 years that a person has cyclothymia there can be no occurrences of major depression, mania, or mixed episodes. Untreated cyclothymia can greatly decrease a person's quality of life, earning power, and family harmony. The illness also has the ability, especially if left untreated, to escalate into a more serious disorder. DSM-IV-TR reports a 15–50% risk for the illness advancing to bipolar I or II.

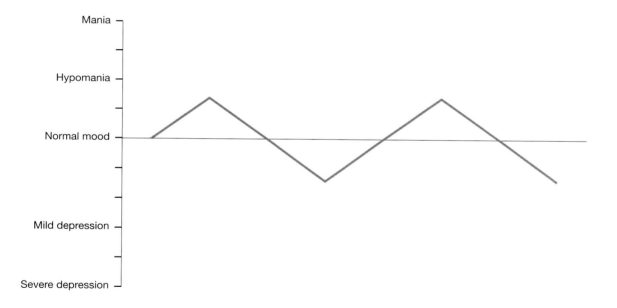

Figure 2.9 Cyclothymia disorder. Adapted from reference 12

When No Diagnosis Fits

When a person does not fully meet the criteria for any of the bipolar disorders, but has symptoms or features of bipolar illness, they are given the diagnosis of bipolar disorder not otherwise specified. DSM-IV-TR provides five examples where the diagnosis would apply.

REFERENCES

1. American Psychiatric Association. Diagnostic and Statistical Manual of Mental Disorders, 4th edn, Text Revision. Washington, DC: American Psychiatric Association, 2000.

2. Taylor EH. Manic–depressive illness. In Ramachandran VS, ed. Encyclopedia of the Human Brain. San Diego: Academic Press, 2002; 2: 745–57.

3. Miklowitz DJ. The Bipolar Disorder Survival Guide. New York: Guilford Press, 2002.

4. Hales D, Hales RE. Caring for the Mind. New York: Bantam Books, 1995.

5. Goldberg JF, Harrow M. Poor-outcome bipolar disorders. In Goldberg JF, Harrow M, eds, Bipolar Disorders: Clinical Course and Outcome. Washington, DC: American Psychiatric Press, 1999: 1–19.

6. Goodwin FK, Jamison KR. Manic–Depressive Illness. New York: Oxford University Press, 1990.

7. Birmaher B. New Hope for Children and Teens with Bipolar Disorder. New York: Three Rivers Press, 2004.

8. Goldberg JF, Kocsis JH. Depression in the course of bipolar disorder. In Goldberg JF, Harrow M, eds. Bipolar Disorders: Clinical Course and Outcome. Washington, DC: American Psychiatric Press, 1999: 129–48.

9. Dubovsky SL, Davies R, Dubovsky A. Mood disorders. In Hales RE, Yudofsky SC, eds. The American Psychiatric Publishing Textbook of Clinical Psychiatry, 4th edn. Washington, DC: American Psychiatric Press, 2003: 439–542.

10. Jamison KR. An Unquiet Mind. New York: Vintage Books, 1995.

11. Torrey EF, Knable MB. Surviving Manic Depression: A Manual on Bipolar Disorder for Patients, Families and Providers. New York: Basic Books, 2002.

12. Mondimore M. Bipolar Disorder: A Guide for Patients and Families. Johns Hopkins Health Book. Baltimore, MD: Johns Hopkins University Press, 1999.

3 Child and Adolescent Bipolar Illness

A small but growing number of studies have been conducted in children and adolescents who develop a bipolar disorder. At how young an age a child can demonstrate symptoms definitively indicating a bipolar disorder rather than other neurobiological problems requires further research, and is controversial within the professional communities.

Parents, however, are advised to keep in mind that the debate is focused more on whether enough evidence exists to declare that a prepubertal child has an adult form of bipolar illness than on whether the symptoms indicate a need for psychiatric intervention. Childhood symptoms often change, overlap, and appear different from those observed in adult mental illness. This complicates, delays, and causes changes in psychiatric diagnosis. Nonetheless, moderate to severe symptoms persisting over time indicate that a child either is on a path toward a major mental health problem or has developed a serious neurobiological disorder.

Diagnostic difficulty in labeling a cluster of childhood symptoms means neither that a youth will fail to benefit from appropriate psychiatric care nor that mental health services should be delayed.

Types of Childhood Bipolar Disorders

- Bipolar I disorder

- Bipolar II disorder

- Cyclothymic disorders (cyclothymia)

- Mood disorders

- Unipolar mood disorders

Attention Deficit Hyperactivity Disorder (ADHD) and Depression: Indicator for Assessment

The National Institute of Mental Health (NIMH) recommends that a child or teen who is depressed along with severe attention deficit hyperactivity disorder (ADHD)-like symptoms, temper outbursts, and mood changes, should be assessed for bipolar illness.

The evaluation is especially urgent if the child is taking medications for the ADHD. Psychostimulant medications prescribed for ADHD can worsen manic symptoms*.

*Source: National Institute of Mental Health (2005). Child and Adolescent Bipolar Disorder: An Update from the National Institute of Mental Health (URL http://www.nimh.gov/publicat/bipolarupdate.cfm)

Additionally, there is evidence that children are at increased risk of early-onset bipolar illness if one or both parents have had a mood disorder or a history of abusing substances[1,2]. Furthermore, children with unipolar depression are at a greater risk for developing a bipolar disorder, and need close observation for early symptoms and indicators of mania or hypomania[3,4]. The lifetime prevalence rate for prepubertal and adolescent bipolar disorders has not been sufficiently studied. However, bipolar I and II and cyclothymic disorders are reported by clinicians as commonly seen in community clinics. The Oregon Adolescent Depression Project reported a lifetime prevalence rate among adolescents of approximately 1%[5]. This study and other findings also suggest that early-onset bipolar disorder may cause more severe symptoms and be a different form of illness than that experienced by older adolescents and adults[6]. Furthermore, some experts and parents believe that a subpopulation of children are born with bipolar symptoms. Parents of bipolar children often report that as infants or toddlers their children cried excessively, were hyperactive, had difficulty being comforted, were highly anxious, and stayed awake far more than other babies[1,2].

Barbara Geller, a leading researcher of child bipolar illness, points out that for children to receive a diagnosis of bipolar disorder they must have symptoms that dimensionally define and frame their manic, depressive, or mixed episodes. A single symptom, such as irritation or agitation, even though a hallmark for both early-onset mania and depression, is not by itself a childhood bipolar disorder[7–9]. Irritation and agitation are seen in numerous child disorders. Therefore, Geller includes children in her bipolar group only if, along with symptoms such as irritation, the child also has an elated mood or grandiosity and fulfills the DSM-IV-TR criteria for mania or hypomania[7–9]. In their clinical work, Demitri and Janice Papolos have observed that children with bipolar disorder tend to show[2]:

(1) Inflexibility;

(2) Oppositional behaviors (Figure 3.1);

(3) Irritability;

(4) An explosive rage that either makes no sense or is far more intense than seen in most children in similar circumstances.

A key factor in diagnosing childhood mania is the context of the behavior. For example, all children are

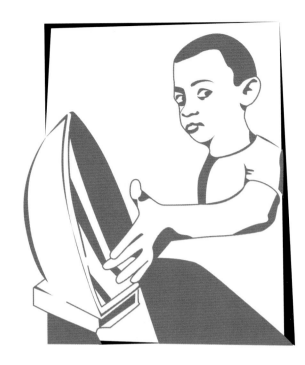

Figure 3.1 Children with mania take risks, and either feel excited by the danger or fail to perceive that they are in danger

excited when going somewhere special. Their behaviors and delight match the environmental context. The manic child, however, can become elated and expansive in situations where other children remain composed. This author worked with a child who, while attending a Cub Scout awards meeting, suddenly started crawling around the room, laughing loudly, and howling like an animal. Similar behaviors also occurred in the boy's classroom and at the home of his parents' friends. Each time the behaviors were different from the conduct of the other children and not in keeping with the environmental context. Derailing the behavior was almost impossible. As the parents tried quieting the laughter and animal sounds, their son became irritated and attempted to hit and scratch the father.

Geller's studies have found that mania in children can cause symptoms similar to those we see in adults, including:

(1) Expanded and elated moods;

(2) Grandiosity beyond the self-perceptions and belief systems of most children;

(3) Extremely decreased sleeping patterns – appearing energetic after staying up all day and having only a few hours of sleep in the evening;

(4) Hypersexuality[9].

Hypersexuality in children may appear in the form of excessive touching of others, touching other people's genitals, masturbation in public or only semi-private locations, sexually suggestive language and body movements, and openly asking to have sex with a peer or adult.

Current research suggests that a majority of children with bipolar illness cycle rapidly between manic, depressive, and mixed episodes. Any combination of episodes can occur from cycle to cycle; that is, as in rapid cycling in adults, the episodes do not have to switch from mania to depression. Unlike in rapid cycling in adults, children tend to have far more than 4–5 episodes in a 12-month period. Almost continuous cycling may occur over days and weeks, making identifying where episodes start and end difficult.

As a result, the cycling can merge into mixed episodes where depression and manic symptoms are experienced simultaneously or one immediately followed by the other (Figures 3.2 and 3.3). This is an extremely dangerous state, since the child may have a high level of energy along with depression and suicidal thoughts, or have no concerns about obvious dangers. As an example, a child in a mixed episode may climb onto a roof or other high point, take no precautions, and hope a fall occurs.

Only a few brain studies using magnetic resonance imaging (MRI), functional MRI (fMRI), and SPECT have been performed on children with bipolar disorders. A review of the literature by DelBello and Kowatch found indications of reduced structural asymmetry of the cerebral hemispheres, deep white-matter hyperintensities, and ventricular abnormalities. However, because of the small sample sizes, the findings must be considered preliminary and to offer no significant conclusions[10]. Studies of adolescents with bipolar disorder using fMRI suggest that abnormalities exist in the subcortical portions of the frontostriatal circuits[11]. Studies by the Stanford Psychiatry Neuroimaging Laboratory found that children with bipolar illness have difficulties with visuospatial working memory. They also documented that young teenagers had greater activation in the prefrontal and paralimbic brain structures than children who had no history of mental illness[12]. In addition, there is evidence that basal thyroid hormone

---

Mania and Children*

- Mania can cause children and adolescents to experience more irritability and destructive outbursts than are generally seen in adults.

- Mania may cause children who normally are not destructive to rip and break home furnishings, punch holes in walls, and spray-paint public walls.

- Rapid cycling that is almost continuous and warps into mixed episodes is more common in children and young adolescents than in adults.

- Even very young children in a manic episode may become hypersexual and proposition other children or adults, excessively touch others, or openly masturbate.

- Grandiosity may cause children to have beliefs such as: they are above the law and have a right to shoplift, they know more than their teachers, they can start a business that will make them rich, they can become wealthy and famous without attending school, or they can attain fame as a musician without talent or knowledge of music.

- Mania can cause a child to go without sleep or sleep only a few hours and appear energetic.

- Risk-taking behaviors can be extremely dangerous; for example, a child may stand on a high ledge with his or her feet partly over the edge, may jump from roofs or other high places, or may try to see how closely he or she can dart in front of a fast-moving car and get out of the way without being hit.

*For additional details on manic symptoms see references 2 and 7.

The Bipolar Depressed Child

A depressed child may show some or all of the following symptoms. An assessment for depression is suggested for any child who, for a week to 10 days, demonstrates any of these behaviors most of each day, or for whom the behaviors continuously appear, disappear, and reappear:

- Frequent complaints of physical problems such as stomach aches, headaches, muscle pain, etc.;

- Isolation, spending an overabundance of time alone;

- Crying for no known reason or showing almost no emotions over situations that upset peers;

- Sad, depressed, or irritable behaviors and communications;

- Change in sleeping (excessive sleeping or not enough sleep);

- Slowed movement or change in coordination;

- Use of alcohol or other substances;

- Change in speech patterns (for example, decreased conversation or responses reflecting agitation and negative feelings);

- Reduced energy and complaints of being tired;

- Problems concentrating, recalling known information, problem-solving issues that the child used to handle routinely, or other signs that 'thinking' and processing information are more difficult;

- Expressions of hopelessness, feeling worthless, or having no chance of things improving;

- Talk and behavior indicating a wish to die, remarks about suicide, discussions about death or life after death.

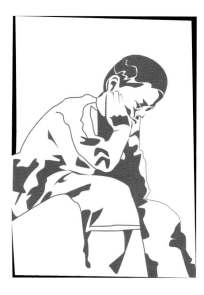

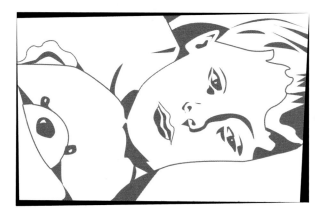

Figure 3.2 Depression can merge with mania, creating a mixed episode. The risk for suicide and destructive behavior to self, others, and property increases during a mixed episode

Figure 3.3 Children with depression often complain of feeling tired. Mania causes the same child to need little or no sleep and appear energetic

levels are abnormal in depressed and manic adolescents[13]. However, until brain and hormonal studies are replicated using more patients and better-controlled research methods, the findings must be considered preliminary and exploratory in nature. Even so, these studies highlight that early brain abnormalities may exist in children and adolescents who have bipolar symptoms and justify the expense of future imaging research.

Childhood bipolar disorder creates a high degree of stress in families. The child is highly unpredictable (Figure 3.4), difficult to manage behaviorally, requires medication supervision, and is stigmatized by portions of society. As a result, both the family and child need ongoing education, support, guidance, and rest.

The family, school system, and mental health treatment team should conduct monthly planning and support meetings. Mental health workers may also take an active role in educating other community systems about bipolar illness and the child's specific support needs. It can be extremely helpful for social workers and nurses to meet routinely with religious leaders, neighbors, and organizational leaders who interact with the child[14]. These individuals often do not understand bipolar disorder or know how best to assist the child and family. Additionally, community agencies must be encouraged to relieve parents from some responsibilities such as child transportation or after-school care. More important, however, the child needs evidence-based treatment.

A recent 2-year study of community interventions in youths who have bipolar disorders discovered that only 47% of the children ($n = 89$) received

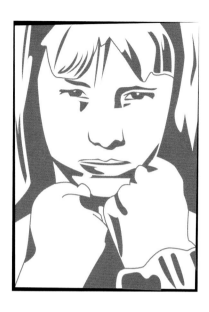

Figure 3.4 Manic episodes can cause children to become extremely aggressive, destroy property, physically fight, and verbally argue for almost no obvious reason

lithium, an anticonvulsant, or a neuroleptic. In addition, the same study found that there was no difference in the rate of recovery between children receiving lithium and those on anticonvulsants. Children on neuroleptics were less likely to recover, although this may reflect a greater severity and more comorbid illness in the children who were prescribed antipsychotic medications.

Antidepressants were given to 29% of the children and 60% received stimulants. Individual, group, and family psychotherapy did not significantly aid in the remission of symptoms[15,16]. Approximately 54%

Antidepressants and Early-Onset Bipolar Depression

- As with adults, antidepressant monotherapy may trigger mania in children and adolescents.

- Particular caution and care are needed when a youth has ADHD symptoms and a family history of bipolar disorder.

- Depressed children must be closely assessed for 'hints' of undiagnosed manic and hypomanic symptoms.

- Depressed children need continuous follow-up and reassessment by mental health professionals for signs of manic and hypomanic behaviors.

- Families of depressed children need to be trained to identify manic and hypomanic behaviors and reminded to watch for hints that the child is cycling.

of the sample received individual and group therapy, and 21% experienced family treatment. Individual and group therapy was associated with less likelihood of recovery. However, the researchers point out that many of these children were treated at psychiatric sites and may, therefore, have had disorders that were more resistant to treatment. Nonetheless, the

study underscores an immediate need for mental health professionals to receive training in assessing and treating childhood bipolar disorders. Additionally, the role of psychotherapy in childhood treatment deserves attention from researchers. In adults, specific forms of supportive and talk therapy appear to assist people in their recovery[17]. Future studies may identify whether young, middle, and older children can benefit from specialized forms of psychotherapy. It is very possible that a child's age along with the severity and phase of the illness determine whether psychotherapy is helpful. Talk and support therapies may not reduce symptoms but may increase the child or family's coping skills or quality of life. However, if any form of treatment is not supported by research, it should not be administered.

Table 3.1 Antidepressants/anxiolytics

	Maximum dose per day	
	Children	Adolescents
Citalopram	40 mg	40 mg
Escitalopram	20 mg	20 mg
Fluvoxamine*	200 mg	200 mg
Fluoxetine*†	20 mg	40 mg
Paroxetine	30 mg	40 mg
Sertraline*	200 mg	200 mg
Venlafaxine	3 mg/kg	225 mg

* Has Food and Drug Administration (FDA) approved labeling for treatment of anxiety disorders in children; *† Has FDA approved labeling for treatment of depression in children.

CHILD MEDICATION TABLES

Tables 3.1–3.4 what generally thought to be the usual maximum doses of common psychotropic medications. Individual patients may require lower or higher doses. When higher dosages are used the doctor will need to document thoroughly the rationale for prescribing a higher dose, and monitor and document carefully all observed and reported treatment responses.

Table 3.2 Antipsychotics

	Maximum dose per day	
	Children	Adolescents
Aripiprazole	15 mg	30 mg
Clozapine	300 mg	600 mg
Haloperidol	10 mg	20 mg
Olanzapine	12.5 mg	20 mg
Quetiapine	No data	600 mg
Risperidone	4 mg	6 mg
Ziprasidone	No data	180 mg

Table 3.3 Attention deficit hyperactivity disorder (ADHD) medications

	Maximum dose per day	
	Children	Adolescents
Amphetamine (Mixed amphetamine salts or dextroamphetamine)	40 mg	40 mg
Atomoxetine	1.8 mg/kg	100 mg
Bupropion	6 mg/kg	400 mg
Clonidine	0.4 mg	0.4 mg
Guanfacine	4 mg	4 mg
Imipramine	5 mg/kg	300 mg
Methylphenidate	60 mg	65 mg
Nortriptyline	3 mg/kg	150 mg

Table 3.4 Mood stabilizers

	Maximum dose per day	
	Children	Adolescents
Carbamazepine*	7 mg/kg	(Max Cs: 12 μg/ml)
Lamotrigine	15 mg/kg (200 mg)	200 mg
Lithium*	30 mg/kg	(Max Cs: 1.2 mmol/l)
Valproic acid* (Divalproex)	20 mg/kg	(Max Cs: 125 μg/ml)

*Maximum (Max) daily dose typically determined by drug serum concentration (Cs) and individual patient tolerability.

Tables 3.1–3.4 are reproduced with permission from the Texas Department of Health Services. The complete document entitled 'Psychotropic Medication Utilization Parameters for Foster Children' is available on the web (http://www.dshs.state.tx.us/mhprograms/ PsychotropicMedicationUtilizationParametersFosterChildren.pdf).

REFERENCES

1. Faedda GL, Baldessanni RJ, Glovinsky IP, Austin NB. Pediatric bipolar disorder: phenomenology and course of illness. Bipolar Disord 2004; 6: 305.

2. Papolos D, Papolos J. The Bipolar Child. The Definitive and Reassuring Guide to Childhood's Most Misunderstood Disorder. New York: Broadway Books, 1999.

3. Wilens TE, Wozniak J. Bipolar disorder in children and adolescents: diagnostic and therapeutic issues. Psychiat Times 2003; 8: 1–8.

4. Geller B, Fox LW, Clark KA. Rate and predictors of prepubertal bipolarity during follow-up of 6- to 12-year-old depressed children. J Am Acad Child Adolesc Psychiatry 1994; 33: 461–8.

5. Lewinsohn P, Seeley JR, Klein D. Bipolar disorder in adolescents. In Geller B, DelBello MP, eds. Bipolar Disorder in Childhood and Early Adolescence. New York: Guilford Press, 2003: 7–24.

6. Geller B, Luby J. Child and adolescent bipolar disorder: a review of the past 10 years. J Am Acad Child Adolesc Psychiatry 1997; 36: 1168–76.

7. Geller B, DelBello MP, eds. Bipolar Disorder in Childhood and Early Adolescence. New York: Guilford Press, 2003.

8. Geller B, Williams M, Zimerman B, et al. Prepubertal and early adolescent bipolarity differentiated from ADHD by manic symptoms, grandiose delusions, ultra-rapid or ultradian cycling. J Affect Disord 1998; 51: 81–91.

9. Geller B, Craney JL, Bolhofner K, et al. Phenomenology and longitudinal course of children with a prepubertal and early adolescent bipolar disorder phenotype. In Geller B, DelBello MP, eds. Bipolar Disorder in Childhood and Early Adolescence. New York: Guilford Press; 2003: 25–50.

10. Delbello MP, Kowatch RA: Neuroimaging in pediatric bipolar disorder. In Geller B, Delbello MP, eds. Bipolar Disorder in Childhood and Early Adolescence. New York: Guilford Press, 2003: 158–74.

11. Blumberg HP, Martin A, Kaufman J, et al: Frontostriatal abnormalities in adolescents with bipolar disorder: preliminary observations from functional MRI. Am J Psychiatry 2003; 160: 1345–7.

12. Chang KD, Adleman N, Menon DK, Reiss V. fMRI of visuospatial working memory in boys with bipolar disorder. Presented at the 49th Annual Meeting of the American Academy of Child and Adolescent Psychiatry, San Francisco, CA, October 2002: Poster.

13. Sokolov STH, Kutcher SP, Joffe RT. Basal thyroid indices in adolescent depression and bipolar disorder. J Am Acad Child Adolesc Psychiatry 1994; 33: 469–75.

14. Taylor EH. Practice methods for working with children who have biologically based mental disorders: a bioecological model. Fam Soc: J Contemp Human Serv 2003; 84: 39–50.

15. Geller B, Craney JL, Bolhofner K, et al. One-year recovery and relapse rates of children with a prepubertal and early adolescent bipolar disorder phenotype. Am J Psychiatry 2001; 158: 303–5.

16. Geller B, Craney JL, Bolhofner K, et al. Two year prospective follow-up of children with a prepubertal and early adolescent bipolar disorder phenotype. Am J Psychiatry 2002; 159: 927–33.

17. Goodwin FK, Jamison KR. Manic–Depressive Illness. New York: Oxford University Press, 1990.

4 Bipolar Disorders and the Changing Brain

From the 1960s through the 1980s, graduate programs and medical schools began not to use the term psychopathology in titles for courses focused on serious mental disorders. Referring to psychiatric problems as pathologies was believed to misrepresent the disorders as being more closely related to biology than was warranted. Today, virtually all major universities and research programs teach that bipolar disorders are illnesses stemming directly from structural and functional brain abnormalities (Figure 4.1).

Thus, psychopathology has been redefined to include the neuropsychiatric or neurobiological brain diseases such as bipolar disorders. Much remains to be learned about the neurophysiology and chemistry of bipolar disorders (Figures 4.2 and 4.3). Nonetheless, studies illustrating that the brains of people with bipolar illnesses differ from those of individuals who have no psychiatric history are rapidly mounting. Mental health research is starting at last to explain why and how bipolar symptoms occur.

While the exact cause of this illness has yet to be pinpointed, scientific findings indicate that bipolar symptoms are best understood as resulting from multiple interacting cellular structures and neurochemical systems that have been significantly altered[1].

Why Neuroscience Imaging Studies Do Not Always Agree

When reading the literature one will discover that imaging studies do not always agree, and sometimes report opposite findings. As an example, one study may report a brain region as enlarged while another claims that the area is smaller than found in normal controls. What the studies have in common is finding that a specific brain structure is significantly different from that found in people with no history of mental illness. Below are some of the reasons that differences in findings occur.

- Different types and models of imaging scanners and blood flow devices are used.

- Technical adjustments to the equipment (calibration) can vary greatly, as can the computer software guiding the equipment.

- Positioning of patients can vary widely.

- The research participants from study to study may all have the same mental disorder, but differ in age, gender, severity of illness, length of time ill, symptoms, medication history, number of episodes, current state of illness, genetic history, etc.

- One study has very specific diagnostic criteria for research participants while a different study accepts people who only broadly meet DSM-IV-TR's diagnostic criteria.

- Many studies simply do not have enough participants.

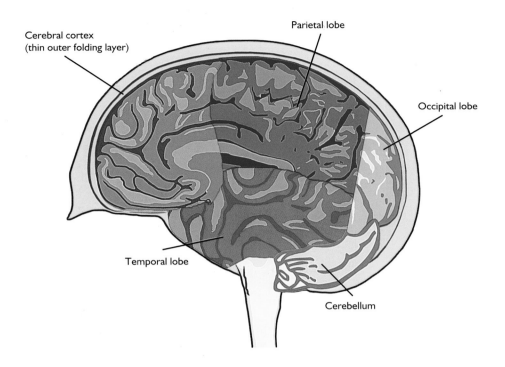

Cerebral cortex
(thin outer folding layer)

Parietal lobe

Occipital lobe

Temporal lobe

Cerebellum

Figure 4.1 Illustration of major brain regions. Bipolar researchers are interested in how the brain's regions play a role in manic and depressive episodes. Because the brain is dynamic and interactive, illustrations of regions and lobes are rather arbitrary. The frontal lobes and cortex provide us with the ability to make social judgments and other executive decisions such as planning and abstract thinking. Language and some long-term memory functions reside in the temporal lobes, while sensory and visual–spatial operations are handled by the parietal lobes. Visual perceptions come through the occipital lobes. In order for the cortex, as an example, to perform executive functions, input is needed from almost every major part of the brain. In the deep center of the brain is the thalamus (not shown), which serves as a way station for almost all information going to the cortex. Without accurate temporal lobe functioning, interpretations of complex visual patterns, spoken language, and long-term memories can be distorted. Abnormalities in the limbic system's amygdala may send forward over- or under-stated emotions. They may also trigger incorrect memories or misperceptions from the hippocampus. The hippocampus may also fail to recall 'maps' that allow a person to navigate easily familiar places and areas. Together, these and other faulty brain interactions create the behaviors and actions that we observe and call manic or depressive symptoms

BRAIN STRUCTURES AND BIPOLAR DISORDERS

The ability to measure and illustrate symbolically deviations in brain functioning between people with bipolar disorders and those with no mental disorder, or differing psychiatric problems, has greatly increased our knowledge and understanding of manic and depressive episodes. Early studies using computed tomography (CT) scans made important but limited contributions to the understanding of bipolar disorders. Neuroimaging using CT and magnetic resonance imaging (MRI) has provided anatomical pictures of the brain. Almost all current anatomical research relies on MRI, which can look

more deeply into the brain and produce images with greater resolution compared with a CT scan. Brain structure is examined through anatomical studies, but brain function is evaluated by assessments that measure and illustrate neuroactivity. The brain is the only organ in the body that is unable to store fuel sources (glycogen, fat, oxygen, etc.). As such, brain cells are intrinsically dependent on the second-by-second delivery of glucose and oxygen to them by the cerebral circulation to maintain activity. Functional neuroactivity can be assessed by measuring metabolism directly (using a radioactive isotope of oxygen or glucose labeled with a radioactive isotope of fluorine – fluorodeoxyglucose), as in positron emission tomography (PET) imaging, or by

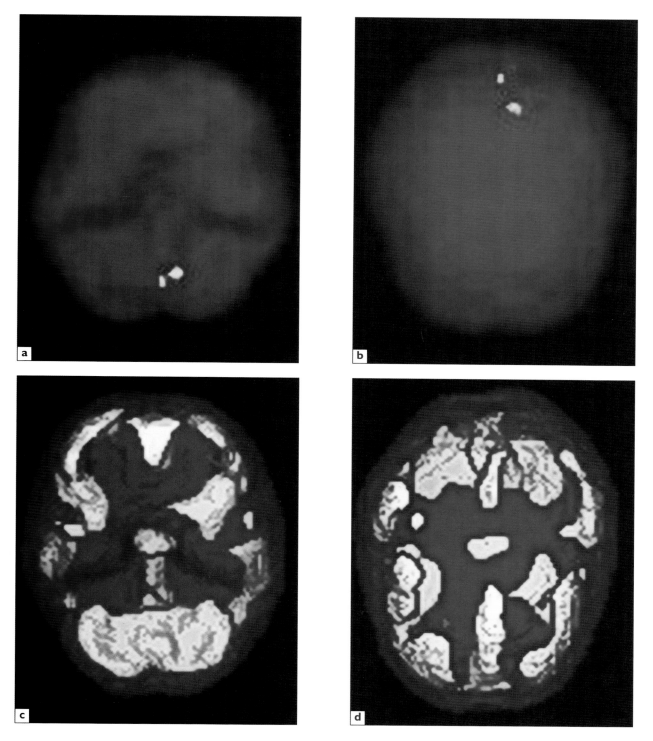

Figure 4.2 Single photon emission computed tomography (SPECT) scans showing a functional comparison of normal brain and a manic episode. Brighter areas represent greater metabolism or rapid functioning. All scans in this figure are reproduced by permission of S. Gregory Hipskind, MD, PhD, and Brain Matters, Inc. (www.brainmattersinc.com).

(a) The inferior brain surface from a person with no history of mental disorders. (b) The superior brain surface from a person with no history of mental disorders. (c) and (d) SPECT scans (threshold set at 85%) of a patient who meets the *Diagnostic and Statistical Manual of Mental Disorders* (DSM-IV-TR) criteria for bipolar I disorder. The bright yellow areas are two standard deviations greater than average. This patient has a long-documented history of bipolar disorder, and was diagnosed by psychiatrists who are not associated with the SPECT scanning laboratory. (c) The inferior surface view of the brain. (d) The superior surface view

measuring metabolism indirectly but reliably by measuring regional cerebral blood flow, as in single photon emission computed tomography (SPECT) imaging. Recent advances in SPECT imaging are now allowing greater resolution than with PET at a much lower cost. How the brain is working in a living person is captured by quantifying the amounts of and locations where either glucose or oxygen is metabolized, or where blood is flowing at higher or lower rates. As brain regions and systems are used for thinking, perceiving, problem-solving, or emotionally

responding, more glucose, oxygen, and blood flow are required in the active sections than in sections that are not directly involved in completing the task.

Brain functioning can be assessed and graphically pictured by computerized regional blood flow monitoring devices, SPECT scans, PET scans, and functional magnetic resonance imaging (fMRI) scans.

In addition to researching the living brain, postmortem neurological studies are also unlocking the secrets of bipolar disorders. This work has been enhanced by improved methods of fixing and

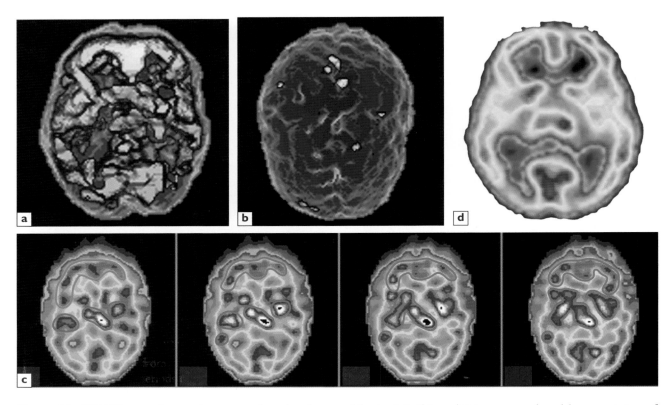

Figure 4.3 SPECT scan of a manic, a normal, and a depressed brain. (a), (b), and (c) are reproduced by permission of William C. Klindt, MD, Silicon Valley Brain SPECT Imaging, Inc., San Jose, California, USA (www.braininspect.com). (d) is reproduced by permission of S. Gregory Hipskind, MD, PhD, and Brain Matters, Inc. (www.brainmattersinc.com).
(a) Manic episode with generalized increased blood flow (overactivity) throughout most brain regions. (b) Normal brain with no history of mental disorder. (c) Depressed brain. (d) Normal brain with no depression. This is a transverse inner brain view of blood flow activity in a person with no mental illness. Together, the two scans (c) and (d) illustrate how depression often increases blood flow and metabolism in limbic areas (circled in red) and decreases activity in the frontal areas (circled in green). The SPECT scan allows one to view functional systems. In these examples we see the brain's internal areas. Hyperperfusion can be seen over most of the overactive brain (yellow to orange colors). This is highly associated with manic episodes (a). The normal brain (b) shows reduced blood flow or activity. The depressed brain (c) has significant hyperperfusion in its thalamolimbic part (circled in red). This region is mostly in the very center of the brain images. The bright yellow, red, and white colors indicate that the blood flow in this area is very rapid. This is a common finding in patients with depression. The four images are cross-sectional transverse views of the same individual. The top of each picture is the front of the brain and the bottom is the back . The slices start 'higher' in the brain and progressively move lower through the brain's thalamolimbic area. In addition to depression the patient also reported problems with anxiety. SPECT studies indicate that anxiety is strongly associated with hyperperfusion in the brain's basal ganglia region. Increased activity is indicated in this person's basal ganglia activity by the white and red markings lateral to the limbic area and circled in red

preserving the brain immediately upon death, better information about donors, more systematic distribution of brain samples to neuroscientists, and the refinement of electronic and computerized microscopes.

BRAIN IMAGING STUDIES

Numerous brain structures appear to play a role in producing bipolar episodes (Table 4.1). An early study at the National Institute of Mental Health's Saint Elizabeth's Hospital Neuropsychiatric Research Program used CT scans to discover that the cerebellum significantly differed in people with bipolar I disorder compared with normal controls[2]. More recently, neuroimaging studies have reported that the brains of individuals with bipolar disorders have structural abnormalities in the amygdala, basal ganglia, cerebellum, hippocampus, prefrontal cortex, temporal lobe, and third ventricle. Additionally, bipolar disorders appear to be associated with a decrease of the brain's gray matter. Ketter and associates reviewed the existing literature and, in addition to the above findings, suggest that there is evidence of sulcal widening and subcortical hyperintensities in patients with bipolar and unipolar depression. They also argue that none of the structural brain findings are consistently associated with symptom severity and other clinical parameters[3]. Bipolar I and II are not thought to be significantly different in hippocampal or temporal lobe size. The lateral ventricle in bipolar I patients may be enlarged compared with that in patients with bipolar II disorder (Figure 4.4)[4]. Additionally, at least one study has reported MRI evidence of ventricular enlargement in adolescents with bipolar disorder[5]. Until further studies are carried out it is currently difficult to draw conclusions about structural changes in adolescents with and without major mental disorders.

Imaging studies document that the amygdala of a bipolar patient differs in size from that in a person with no psychiatric history. Conflicts remain, however, in that both increased and decreased volume measurements have been reported. For example, separate studies led by Brambilla[7], Strakowski[8], and Altshuler[9] found the amygdala of people with bipolar disorders to be enlarged, while Pearlson and associates[10] reported the opposite. Additionally, an MRI study of adolescents and adults found that, compared with normal controls with no history of mental illness, people with bipolar I disorder had a significant reduction in amygdala and hippocampal volume[11]. Other studies have documented that patients with bipolar disorder have less gray matter in the prefrontal cortex area of the brain[12,13].

In at least one study comparing brain regions of twins with bipolar I disorder and twins with schizophrenia, the subjects with bipolar illness had less structural damage to the hippocampus–amygdala than those with schizophrenia[14]. Identical results were reported in a study comparing people with schizophrenia, bipolar disorders, or no history of mental illness. A greater decrease in hippocampal and amygdala size was found in subjects with schizophrenia than in people with bipolar I disorder or in normal controls[15]. Other structural differences have been demonstrated between schizophrenia and bipolar disorders. MRI indicates that greater temporal lobe abnormalities and less gray matter are found in the left posterior superior temporal gyrus of

Table 4.1 Functions of key brain regions relating to bipolar illness

Cortex	Amygdala	Hippocampus	Hypothalamus
Abstract thinking:	Emotions:	Memories:	Appetite for food
Planning	Rage	Access to most brain signals	Sexual arousal
Conscious thought	Fear	More than just memory –	Body temperature
Judgment	Pleasure	acquires knowledge or information	Sleep cycle
Abstract thinking and insight	Needed for recognition of	from interactions between person	
Hearing	emotions in facial expressions	and social world	
Vision	Helps process emotionally important		
Taste	information communicated in social		
settings by others			

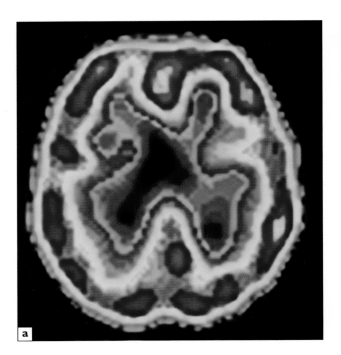
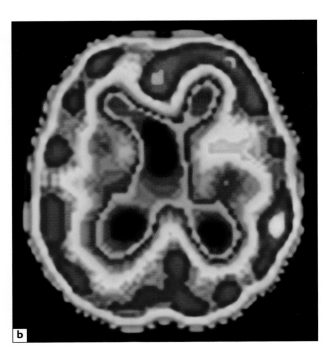

Figure 4.4 (a) SPECT scan of 7-year-old boy with enlarged ventricles. Reproduced by permission of S. Gregory Hipskind, MD, PhD, and Brain Matters, Inc. (www.brainmattersinc.com). The child has a history of resistance to medication treatment. Symptoms include problems regulating mood, paranoid thoughts, and possible auditory and visual hallucinations. Current diagnosis is bipolar I disorder. Because of the enlarged ventricles, mood swings, and possible thought disorder, an alternative diagnosis of schizoaffective disorder must also be considered. (b) Same child with enlarged ventricles, different resolution

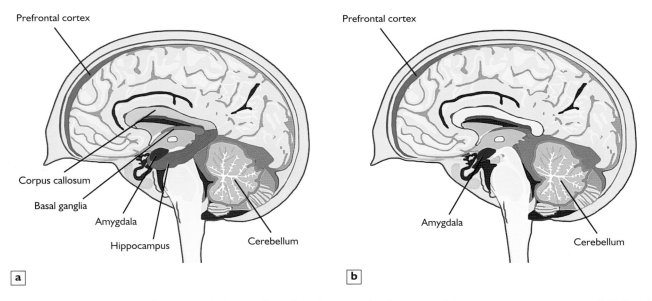

Figure 4.5 (a) Location of anatomical abnormalities found in unipolar depression. Magnetic resonance imaging (MRI) and postmortem research has found unipolar depression to be associated with abnormalities in the brain regions indicated. Functional abnormalities are found in unipolar and bipolar disorders, but unlike anatomical deviations they do not differentiate one disorder from the other[6]. (b) Location of anatomical abnormalities found in bipolar disorders

people with first-episode schizophrenia than in patients with a first-episode bipolar disorder[16]. It is currently unclear whether individuals with bipolar illness have an overall decrease in the region's volume[10,17]. If the lobe's size is diminished, it does not occur as dramatically as seen in schizophrenia. This overall greater level of damage may partially explain why schizophrenia often decreases a person's life skills even after the psychotic episode has passed, while people with bipolar disorder generally return to their pre-illness level of functioning after an episode. Nonetheless, these areas appear often to be anatomically changed in bipolar disorders. Temporal lobe studies in bipolar patients have produced mixed results.

Individuals with schizophrenia also have a more pronounced sulcal region than that of bipolar patients[18]. While mood disorders have been associated with increased sulcal volume, the enlargement most often does not correlate with polarity, and the findings' statistical magnitude only ranges from moderate to weak[3]. Finally, unlike schizophrenia, periventricular deep white-matter hyperintensities (WMH) or lesions generally do not appear in unipolar and bipolar disorders except in older people who develop a late-onset mood disorder. Postmortem studies have documented that the WMH findings in aged patients are more often related to cerebrovascular disease than to bipolar or unipolar illness[6,19–20].

Evidence is growing that the corpus callosum does not change in area, thickness, or length, but may take on a different shape in patients with bipolar illness[14,21]. The change in shape appears to be caused by increased ventricular size[14]. As brain regions such as the ventricles increase in size, pressure can cause other structures to be reshaped or to decrease in total volume. Researchers estimate that ventricular enlargement occurs in 10–31% of patients with bipolar disorders[22]. Bipolar illness may cause progressive changes within the brain. A research group headed by Strakowski compared major brain regions of people experiencing their first bipolar episode with those who had numerous manic episodes. The multiple-episode group had significantly larger lateral ventricles than those of the first-episode group but did not differ in measurements of the striatum. However, the striatum differed significantly between first-episode bipolar patients and control subjects. A statistically non-significant trend indicating a difference in striatum volume was also

reported between the multiple-episode group and healthy controls[23]. The multiple-episode patients' average lateral ventricular volume was 122% greater than that of the first-episode group[23]. There have also been examples of early cerebellar abnormalities occurring in bipolar and unipolar disorders[24,25]. It is speculated, but not yet proven, that cerebellar changes may trigger future abnormalities in catecholamines and the functioning of limbic and cortical areas as bipolar illness progresses[20]. While additional studies are needed, these findings suggest that, over time, a bipolar disorder may cause, or be caused by, degenerating brain structures. The research also illustrates that brain abnormalities exist from the very first bipolar episode, and that some, but not all, of the affected structures may continue to change shape or decrease in size.

No basal ganglia shape or volume changes were found in identical twins discordant for bipolar disorder[14]. Similar negative results have also been reported by a number of researchers[26–29]. This is interesting, because basal ganglia abnormalities are commonly found in people with unipolar depression. Anatomically, bipolar disorders are more associated with changes in the amygdala, temporal cortex, cerebellum, third ventricle, structures near the third ventricle, and the prefrontal cortex, while patients with unipolar major depressive episodes more often have abnormalities in their basal ganglia, frontal cortex, cerebellum, and hippocampus[6,23,30] (Figure 4.5). Both bipolar and unipolar patients with strong family histories of mood disorders have reduced glial cells in the subgenual prefrontal cortex[31].

BRAIN METABOLISM AND BIPOLAR DISORDERS

The secrets of bipolar illness are rapidly being unlocked by machines and computers that allow us to measure and graphically view how a living brain functions (Figure 4.6). SPECT, PET, and fMRI scans illustrate numerous changes in brain functioning or metabolism of patients with bipolar disorder. A small number of studies suggest that, unlike in unipolar depression, bipolar patients have slowed blood flow or glucose metabolism throughout their major brain regions[22,32]. Further studies are needed before it can be assumed that bipolar illness is uniquely associated with a global reduction in metabolic rates.

Conflicting and limited results have emerged from PET and SPECT studies of mania.

Nonetheless, there is evidence that patients experiencing a hypomanic episode produce increased global cerebral metabolism compared with patients who have either bipolar depression or mixed episodes (Figure 4.7). However, this significant difference disappears when hypomania rates are compared with global cerebral metabolism of individuals with no mental illness[3]. A 1997 investigation using PET suggests increased glucose metabolism in the subgenual prefrontal cortex of manic patients compared with normal controls and patients with bipolar and unipolar depression[12]. The metabolism

rates are thought to differ during manic episodes because of findings indicating that gray-matter volume in this region has decreased[33]. Additionally, metabolism in the subgenual prefrontal cortex for depressed patients was significantly slower than for the normal controls[12]. Reduced glucose metabolism has also been found in the medial temporal subcortical region of bipolar depressed patients[34–36]. Future research may validate current small studies showing that metabolism decreases in the frontal and temporal cortical regions when a patient is depressed, and increases during a manic episode (Figure 4.8)[37].

The most consistent finding by SPECT and other instruments has been a pattern of reduced

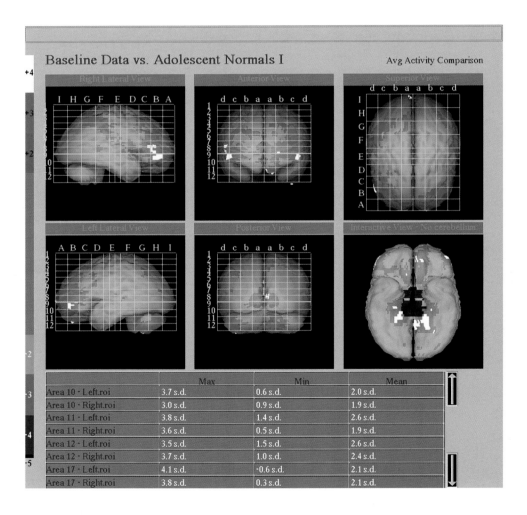

Figure 4.6 Comparison of normal and abnormal Talairach Brain. These images are of an adolescent having a manic episode, produced using SPECT software to perform Talairach Brain scanning measurements. The Talairach Brain refers to an atlas of brain coordinates that can be used to create a computer grid over the scanned brain. The system was developed by Dr Jean Talairach. In this figure the numbers along the grid's side correspond with standard Brodman mapping areas used by doctors, neuroscientists, and other researchers. The grid allows researchers to compare brain regions across subjects. Most important, when combined with a database containing measurements from normal subjects, the Talairach Brain can be used to evaluate specific brain areas of a single patient compared with standardized or expected data from normal subjects

functioning or slowed metabolism in the frontal cortex in both unipolar and bipolar disorders[36,38–45]. This functional slowing combined with frontal anatomical changes partially explains why people with depression and mania have difficulty in performing ordinary mental activities. The region of the brain responsible for discovering alternative solutions, reasoning, maintaining attention, working memory, perceiving and understanding abstract issues, and executing moral and social judgments has been structurally and functionally altered[1]. Social cognitive skills of this nature are sometimes referred to as the brain's executive functions. Patients with schizophrenia usually exhibit far more extensive frontal structural damage and slowed metabolism than those with a bipolar disorder. Consequently, bipolar patients have fewer deficits in their executive functions than do patients with moderate to severe schizophrenia. Furthermore, between depressive or manic episodes, many people with bipolar disorder regain their pre-illness level of social cognitive and problem-solving skills.

Unfortunately, this is less true for people with schizophrenia. Even after a psychotic episode dissipates, patients with schizophrenia or schizoaffective disorder often demonstrate a reduced ability to think abstractly, plan, solve problems, or adequately perform other tasks requiring a high level of sustained frontal activity. During periods of severe depression, mania, or psychosis, a person with bipolar disorder may appear to have executive frontal skills that are as dysfunctional as those seen in patients with schizophrenia or schizoaffective disorder.

Neuropsychologists use the Wisconsin Card Sort to assess the brain's frontal executive functioning. When not in the midst of an episode, patients with bipolar disorder normally perform better on the instrument than those with schizophrenia, and often as well as individuals with no history of mental illness. However, this separation disappears when a person has moderate to severe symptoms of mania. Manic episodes cause Wisconsin Card Sort scores to decrease to a point not significantly different from

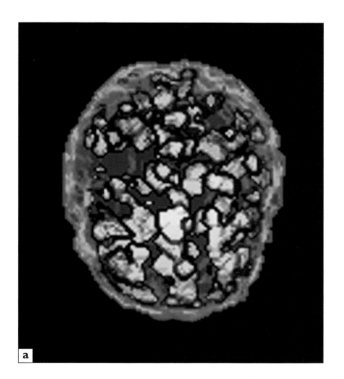
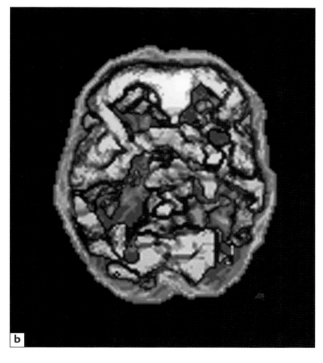

Figure 4.7 Hypomanic episode. Reproduced by permission of William C. Klindt, MD, Silicon Valley Brain SPECT Imaging, Inc. San Jose, California, USA (www.braininspect.com). (a) This is a SPECT scan of a child diagnosed with bipolar I disorder in a hypomanic episode. The image shows increased activity throughout much of the child's brain (orange and yellow areas), but not to the degree found during a manic episode. (b) Compared with mania, the blood flow and metabolism are not as great in a number of regions, but particularly in the frontal areas

results found in studies of schizophrenia[46]. There is some evidence that when acute mania is present, none of the neuropsychological measures robustly differentiate bipolar disorders from schizophrenia[47].

During bipolar depressive episodes without psychotic features, individuals perform much better on cognitive measures than those with schizophrenia[48]. Nevertheless, neuropsychological testing, including fMRI and SPECT findings, demonstrates that bipolar depression is associated with a decrease in the brain's frontal executive skills. Depression causes performance deficits on measures of problem solving and attention[49]. After reviewing the available research literature, Bearden and colleauges state that the frontal slowing observed in chronic bipolar illness does not appear to be significantly related to medication side-effects[22]. The authors caution that their conclusions could be wrong for patients who take multiple medications or a higher than normal dosage. The impact of polydrug therapy and higher-dosage treatments on cognitive skills requires close attention, ongoing assessments, and better-controlled studies[22].

BIPOLAR DISORDERS AND NEUROTRANSMITTERS

Bipolar disorders occur at least in part by complex interactions among neurotransmitters[1]. Researchers have historically linked bipolar disorders to dopamine, serotonin (5-hydroxytryptamine), norepinephrine (noradrenaline), GABA (γ-aminobutyric acid), and glutamate (Figures 4.9–4.15). In addition to the above transmitters, researchers have found changes in acetylcholine and opiate neurotransmitters[50]. In the late 1950s and throughout the 1960s, it was thought that bipolar depression was triggered as norepinephrine decreased and that manic symptoms were dependent on increased levels of dopamine. This became known as the catecholamine hypothesis, because both of the identified neurotransmitters were classified as catecholamines[1,51]. Unlike the early single-neurotransmitter hypotheses, we now know that no single neurochemical or brain process is the primary factor in bipolar disorders. This is particularly true in light of the fact that the brain's transmitting chemicals and electrical processes do

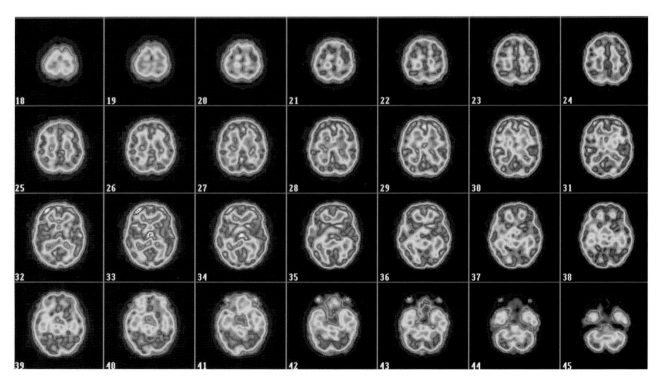

Figure 4.8 Example of manic episode activity captured over time by SPECT technology. Reproduced by permission of William C. Klindt, MD, Silicon Valley Brain SPECT Imaging, Inc., San Jose, California, USA (www.braininspect.com). This is a transverse view of a patient with bipolar disorder. The red and white areas indicate significant hyperperfusion. Increased blood flow and metabolism occur throughout the brain as the manic episode increases. Observe how the rate of activity changes slightly across the scans until the dramatic decrease at the end of the cycle

not act in a vacuum. The brain's principal communication mechanisms are in a coordinated dancing interplay with numerous subtypes of neuroreceptors, second-messenger mediators, and regional brain structures. For example, there are nine or more different types of serotonin receptors spread throughout the brain[52], which serve as docking ports and electrically stimulate signals to be carried down their extended hair-like axons.

Small microsurges and reductions in the amounts of neurotransmitters can change how the brain's receptors function. In recent year, professionals and the general public have become aware that medications can control or inhibit selective serotonin and norepinephrine reuptake. Reuptake is the process used by the brain to store or eliminate neurochemicals remaining after signals are transmitted from one cell to another. Therefore, if depression is exhibited when the volume of a specific neurotransmitter is low, it is useful to prevent or inhibit the uptake process[1]. However, changes in the brain's chemistry can be altered by numerous factors other than the reuptake process. There may be an over- or underproduction of neurotransmitters, chemicals can fail to break down properly, or the receiving neurons may contain too many or too few receptors. Receptors are located on the surfaces of neurons, and changes in their number modify how chemical signals are gathered and processed.

How antidepressants work continues to be a topic of research and debate. We know that all antidepressants interact with one or more monoamine neurotransmitter receptors or enzymes. In general, antidepressants block monoamine reuptake, α_2 receptors, or the enzyme monoamine oxidase (MAO). Most antidepressants currently on the market appear to block the reuptake system[54]. Lithium, which also reduces depression for many

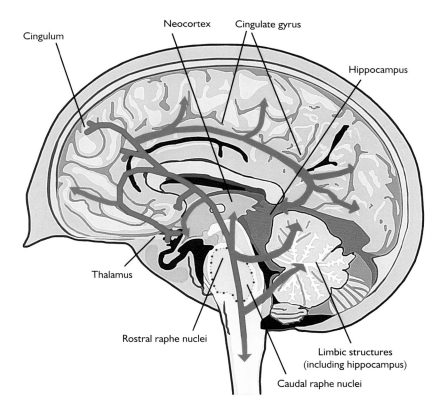

Figure 4.9 Example of serotonin pathway. Serotonin (5-hydroxytryptamine) is found in much of the brain. The neurotransmitter winds from deep in the brain to the outer parts of the frontal cortex. Serotonin neuron receptors are found in the major brain regions associated with bipolar illness such as the limbic system (especially the amygdala, hippocampus, and cingulate gyrus), frontal lobes, frontal cortex, and brain stem (pons and medulla – dotted region). Additionally, serotonin moves through the thalamus, which is found almost in the center of the brain. The thalamus is important in mood disorders because it receives, and partially processes, sensations created by key brain regions and forwards the interacting messages to the frontal lobes and cortex, where they are processed into 'executive' functions and behaviors. Modified from reference 52, with permission

people with a bipolar disorder, is thought to work by changing the brain's second-messenger systems. Just how this takes place is yet to be discovered. Some believe that lithium alters the ability of G proteins to change biological properties into electrical voltage (transducer) once a neurotransmitter has occupied the receptor. There is also the possibility that lithium works by changing enzymes that interact with specific second-messenger systems[54]. Similarly, it is uncertain how valproic acid and carbamazepine (see Chapter 6) help to reduce bipolar symptoms. Valproic acid (Depakote®) may, among other things, inhibit sodium and calcium channels[54]. This is thought both to reduce GABA activity and to lessen glutamate's excitatory actions. Carbamazepine, an anticonvulsant, is hypothesized to enhance the inhibiting actions of GABA by altering the brain's

sodium and potassium channels. Lamotrigine is also thought to block sodium channels and inhibit glutamate's excitatory actions[54]. As discussed in Chapter 6, lamotrigine and valproic acid have provided better results in treating bipolar symptoms than those obtained with carbamazepine.

Researchers are currently interested in discovering how medications influence gene expression. Depression is hypothesized to be associated with abnormal neurotransmitter-inducible gene expression. That is, in addition to other actions caused by antidepressants on receptors and enzymes, they will at some point activate or inactivate key genes. Furthermore, antidepressants may fail to help some patients because the drugs are unable to stimulate the required genetic responses[54].

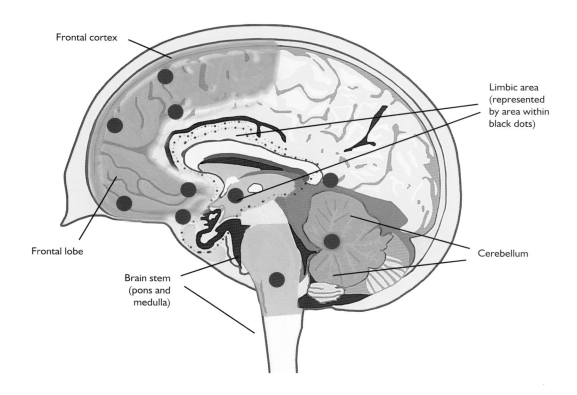

Figure 4.10 Norepinephrine pathways thought to influence bipolar illness. Norepinephrine (noradrenaline) is a key neurotransmitter related generally to mood. It also has a role in arousal and memory. An excess of norepinephrine is associated with manic episodes, while depressive episodes are thought to relate to abnormally reduced quantities of the neurochemical. The red dots illustrate how norepinephrine pathways come from the brain stem to the cerebellum, through much of the limbic system and into the frontal lobes and frontal cortex. These brain regions are known to be involved in both manic and depressive episodes. The cerebellum has not been discussed elsewhere in this chapter. Damage to this part of the brain can, among other things, result in difficulties with memory, retrieving the right word, and controlling rapid sequential movement that requires accurate timing (such as tapping a rhythm). In differing forms these problems are often observed in both depressive and manic episodes. Adapted from reference 54, with permission

Modern imaging, brain metabolism, and post-mortem studies have documented abnormalities in the dopaminergic, serotonergic, and noradrenergic systems. As an example, bipolar patients with psychosis, compared with bipolar patients with no history of psychotic symptoms, have a greater potential for striatal dopamine (D2) binding[55]. A review of the literature by Soares and Innis reveals that postmortem brain findings indicate serotonergic problems in both bipolar and unipolar depression. The authors also found evidence from postmortem studies of increased noradrenergic turnover in cortical areas[6]. PET research indicates changes in serotonin receptors for depressed patients. There is increasing evidence from *in vivo* studies of rather constant abnormalities in the serotonergic and noradrenergic systems. Future research may discover that the severity of these receptor alterations can predict vulnerability for recurrent episodes[56]. However, as pointed out by Mayberg and colleagues[50], it is not yet clear whether these receptor alterations are primarily related to mood disorders.

CONCLUSION

Many of the brain studies are small, and contradictions occur for a number of findings. Still, when taken as a whole, bipolar disorders appear to be associated with and influenced by abnormalities in the brain's anatomical structure, glucose metabolism, and neurotransmitter and second-messenger systems. Furthermore, there is growing evidence that all anti-depressants stimulate critical genes to activate or inactivate. Studies of the brain are not only redefining bipolar illness and underscoring that it is a neurobiological disorder, but also opening doors for the discovery of new medications and treatments. The journey to discover how medications work has begun. Once this mystery is solved, drugs to attack symptoms more effectively and cause fewer side-effects will be developed.

One of the hoped-for developments in clinical work is that brain scans will provide definitive diagnoses of mental disorders (Figure 4.16). Today, scans and glucose metabolism can ensure that symptoms attributed to a mental disorder are not originating from tumors and other hidden abnormalities. They may also be helpful as a means of confirming difficult diagnoses and tracking neurological changes over time.

Currently, however, people should not think of MRI, fMRI, PET, or SPECT as primary diagnostic instruments. No accepted national or international standard has been established for interpreting their findings. More important, insufficient studies have

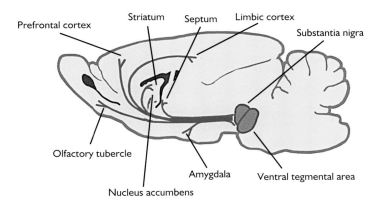

Figure 4.11 The midbrain dopamine system of the rat. Serotonin, norepinephrine, and dopamine are the primary neurotransmitters associated with bipolar illness. All three neurochemicals have pathways through the limbic system. Dopamine is associated with motor control, pleasure-seeking activities, and goal-directed behaviors. There is a strong association between psychotic symptoms and increased dopamine. The primary pathways in the human brain for dopamine are[1]: substantia nigra ↔ ventral tegmental area ↔ amygdala ↔ tuberoinfundibular dopamine system ↔ nucleus accumbens (ventral striatum) ↔ striatum (caudate nucleus, putamen, and globus pallidus) ↔ frontal cortex. The rat's midbrain dopamine pathways are pictured here. Dopamine is associated with reward-seeking behaviors in rats and pleasure in humans. Additionally, the rat pathways involve many of the same brain regions found in the human primary dopamine tracks. This has allowed the rat to be used as a model for studying depression and psychosis in bipolar disorders and schizophrenia[2]. Modified from reference 52, with permission

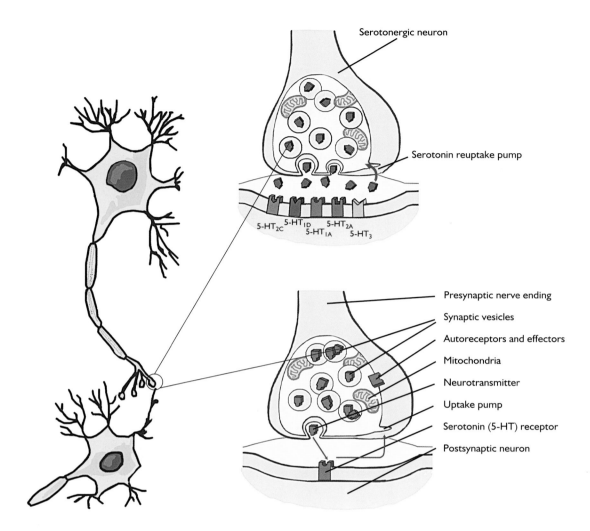

Figure 4.12 Illustration of a serotonergic neuron and synaptic cleft. Neurons are responsible for the brain's intercellular communications. A neuron's parts include a cell body, a long linking tube-like structure known as an axon, and hair-like structures called dendrites. Dendrites intercept impulses from other nerve cells. The intercepted impulse travels electrically along the axon. When electrical messages can go no further down the axon, neurochemical molecules are released. The molecules transport the coded messages to the next receiving neuron. It is the responsibility of neurotransmitter chemicals to transfer impulses (messages) across a microspace separating one neuron from another. This small gap between neurons is called the synaptic cleft. Adapted from reference 53, with permission

Figure 4.13 *(top of opposite page)*   Illustration of a noradrenergic synapse and SNRI uptake site. Serotonin and norepineph-rine (noradrenaline) are closely related neurotransmitters that affect a person's mood. In unipolar depression selective norepinephrine reuptake inhibitor (SNRI) medications can decrease symptoms when selective serotonin reuptake inhibitor (SSRI) drugs have not been effective. The SNRI uptake site is illustrated here. However, even though SNRIs function differ-ently from SSRIs they are not recommended as a monotherapy for bipolar disorders. When used for decreasing bipolar depression, the SNRIs are to be coupled with lithium or an anticonvulsant medication. All antidepressants are considered a third line of defense. Mood stabilizers are the first choice for decreasing depressive symptoms, followed by atypical antipsy-chotic drugs, and finally antidepressants in combination with a mood stabilizer. The use of two or more types of medication for treating bipolar disorders has become standard practice when a single mood stabilizer alone fails to reduce symptoms[1,2]. Modified from reference 53, with permission

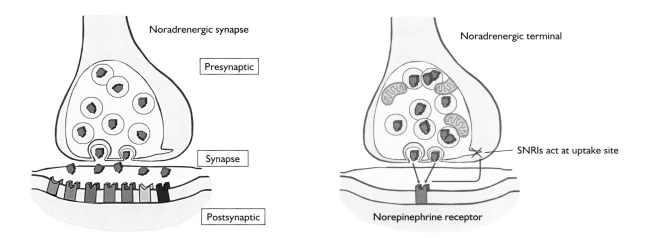

Figure 4.13

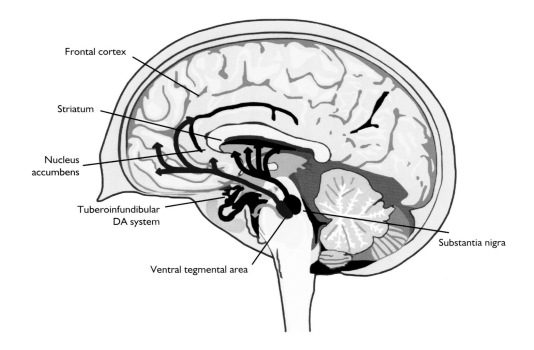

Figure 4.14 Dopaminergic pathways. Dopamine is a multipurpose neurotransmitter responsible for, among other things, pleasure–reward-seeking behaviors, physical movement, and regulation of body temperature. It has long been known that an overproduction of dopamine is associated with psychosis. Antipsychotic medications are thought to work by blocking D_2 receptors in the mesolimbic and mesocortical tracts[1]. However, if these receptors are overly blocked, parkinsonian movements will occur. In addition to psychosis, dopamine can also play an important interactive role in the cause of depression. Depression that primarily relates to dopamine receptors does not respond to SSRI interventions. The substantia nigra pathways illustrated in black strongly influence much of the limbic system, including the striatum. In addition, Parkinson's disease deteriorates substantia nigra neurons' axons and body cells. The arrows in brown illustrate dopamine moving from the ventral tegmental area into the nucleus accumbens and frontal cortex. The green arrow indicates a pathway to the amygdala, while the blue arrows at the lower left trace the tuberoinfundibular dopamine system[1]. The primary dopamine tracts interact with the major regions known to be associated with both manic and depressive episodes. Furthermore, medications that block dopamine receptors, such as haloperidol, often decrease mania and psychosis while drugs such as cocaine stimulate dopamine production and can induce manic behaviors. Modified from reference 52, with permission

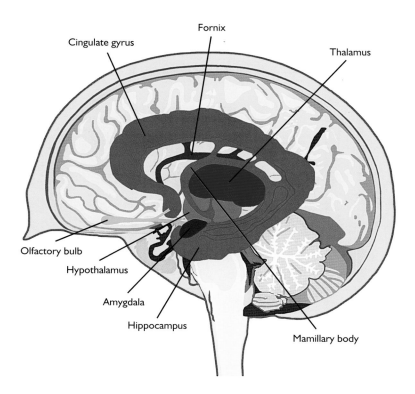

Figure 4.15 Bipolar illness is related to abnormal interactions throughout the brain. Illustrated here are key brain areas thought to interact and play important roles in forming symptoms related to depression and mania. The limbic system (cingulate gyrus, amygdala, hippocampus, etc.) and frontal areas are of particular importance. Together they are responsible for, among other things, memory, emotion, interpreting social meaning, internal and external perceptions, planning, abstract thinking, and judgment. Additionally, serotonin, norepinephrine, and dopamine neurotransmitter pathways interlace throughout the areas (see the neurotransmitter pathway diagrams). Furthermore, psychosis in schizophrenia and bipolar disorders is strongly associated with these same brain regions and neurotransmitters. Greater limbic and frontal abnormalities, however, are found in schizophrenia than in bipolar illness

been conducted to guide an accurate diagnosis. Many of the existing studies consist of very small samples and have not been replicated. For example, as reported in this chapter, one study indicated that people with a bipolar disorder often have enlarged ventricles, but patients and families should keep in mind that the same finding will occur in people with no mental disorder. It simply will not be found as often as it is in people with mental illnesses such as bipolar disorder, schizophrenia, or schizoaffective disorders. Nevertheless, our understanding of the brain and mental disorders is changing because of these instruments. The instruments available today serve a legitimate and increasingly important clinical purpose when used for research, baseline brain functioning and structure documentation, assurance that mental illness symptoms are not secondary to other neurological problems, and support for difficult diagnoses.

REFERENCES

1. Taylor EH. Manic-depressive illness. In Ramachandran VS, ed. Encyclopedia of the Human Brain. San Diego: Academic Press, 2002; 2: 745–57.

2. Weinberger D, DeLisi LE, Perman GP, et al. Computed tomography in schizophreniform and other acute psychiatric disorders. Arch General Psychiatry 1982; 39: 778–83.

3. Ketter TA, George MS, Kimbrell TA, et al. Neuroanatomical models and brain imaging studies. In Young LT, Joffe RT, eds. Bipolar Disorder: Biological Models and Their Clinical Applications. New York: Marcel Dekker, 1997: 179–217.

4. Hauser P, Matochik J, Altschuler LL, et al. MRI-based measurements of temporal lobe and ventricular structures in patients with bipolar I and bipolar II disorders. J Affect Disord 2000; 60: 25–32.

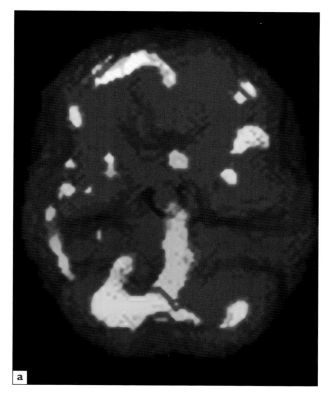
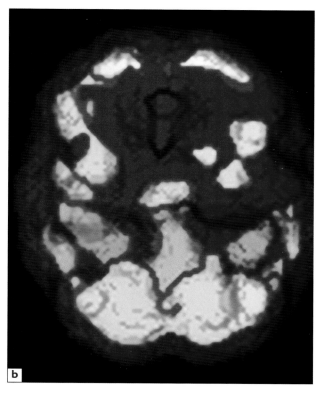

Figure 4.16 SPECT scan, bipolar with comorbid attention deficit hyperactivity disorder (ADHD). Reproduced by permission of S. Gregory Hipskind, MD, PhD, and Brain Matters, Inc., (ww.brainmattersinc.com). (a) Left lateral view. (b) Posterior view. The images illustrate how brain studies have the ability to identify specific functioning related to comorbid disorders. A SPECT scan with concentration test was performed in a preteen child diagnosed with bipolar illness and ADHD. Notice how blood flow is decreased in the frontal cortex and frontal lobe regions, as well as areas of part of the temporal lobe region. This is a consistent pattern found in youths with comorbid bipolar disorder and ADHD. Interestingly, decreased metabolism in the temporal rather than the frontal region has been reported by one study as a more robust indicator of comorbid ADHD in children and young teens[57]. However, the study requires replication using a larger sample and children with better-documented comorbid mood disorders before the findings can be used diagnostically. Use of SPECT imaging and other computerized technologies can greatly help a treatment team's decision-making process. The overlapping symptoms of bipolar illness and ADHD can be indistinguishable even to trained observers when only standard non-imaging assessment methods are used. SPECT cannot stand alone as a diagnostic instrument; it can, however, provide important information that is unobtainable from interviews, psychological testing, or observation

5. Friedman L, Finding RL, Kenny JT, et al. An MRI study of adolescent patients with either schizophrenia or bipolar disorder as compared to healthy control subjects. Biol Psychiatry 1999; 46: 78–88.

6. Soares JC, Innis RB. Brain imaging findings in bipolar disorder. In Soares JC, Gershon S, eds. Bipolar Disorders: Basic Mechanisms and Therapeutic Implications. New York: Marcel Dekker, 2000.

7. Brambilla P, Harenski K, Nicoletti M, et al. MRI investigation of temporal lobe structures in bipolar patients. J Psychiatr Res 2003; 37: 287–95.

8. Strakowski SM, DelBello MP, Sax KW, et al. MRI brain structual abnormalities in bipolar disorder. Arch Gen Psychiatry 1999; 56: 254–60.

9. Altshuler LL, Bartzokis G, Grieder T, et al. Amygdala enlargement in bipolar disorder and hippocampal reduction in schizophrenia: an MRI study demonostrating neuroanatomic specificity. Arch Gen Psychiatry 1998; 55: 663–4.

10. Pearlson GD, Barta PE, Powers RE, et al. Ziskind-Somerfeld Research Award 1996. Medial and superior temporal gyral volumes and cerebral asymmetry in bipolar disorder. Biol Psychiatry 1997; 41: 1–14.

11. Blumberg HP, Kaufman J, Martin A, et al. Amygdala and hippocampal volumes in adolescents and adults with bipolar disorder. Arch Gen Psychiatry 2003; 60: 1201–8.

12. Drevets WC, Price JL, Simpson JR Jr, et al. Subgenual prefrontal cortex abnormalities in mood disorders. Nature 1997; 386: 824–7.

13. Lopez-Larson MP, DelBello MP, Zimmerman ME, et al. Regional prefrontal gray and white matter abnormalities in bipolar disorder. Biol Psychiatry 2002; 52:93–100.

14. Torrey EF, Bowler AE, Taylor EH, Gottesman II. Schizophrenia and Manic Depressive Disorder. The Biological Roots of Mental Illness as Revealed by the Landmark study of Identical Twins. New York: Basic Books, 1994.

15. Altshuler LL, Bartzokis G, Grieder T, et al. An MRI study of temporal lobe structures in men with bipolar disorder or schizophrenia. Biol Psychiatry 2000; 48: 147–62.

16. Hirayasu Y, Shenton ME, Salisbury DF, et al. Lower left temporal lobe MRI volumes in patients with first-episode schizophrenia compared with psychotic patients with first-episode affective disorder and normal subjects. Am J Psychiat 1998; 155: 1384–91.

17. Hauser I, Altschuler LL, Berrettini W, et al. Temporal lobe measurements in primary affective disorder by magnetic resonance imaging. J Neuropsychiatry Clin Neurosci 1989; 1: 128–34.

18. Elkis H, Friedman L, Wise A, Meltzer HY. Meta-analysis of studies of ventricular enlargement and cortical sulcal prominence in mood disorders: comparisons with controls or patients with schizophrenia. Arch Gen Psychiatry 1995; 52: 735–46.

19. Awad IA, Johnson PC, Spectsler RJ, et al. Incidental subcortical lesions identified on magnetic resonance imaging in the elderly, II: postmortem pathological correlations. Stroke 1986, 17: 1090–7.

20. Chimowitz MI, Estes ML, Furlan AJ, et al. Further observations on the pathology of subcortical lesions identified on magnetic resonance imaging. Arch Neurol 1992, 49: 747–52.

21. Frumin M, Golland P, Kikinis R, et al. Shape differences in the corpus callosum in first-episode schizophrenia and first-episode psychotic affective disorder. Am J Psychiatry 2002; 159: 866–8.

22. Bearden CE, Hoffman KM, Cannon TD. The neuropsychology and neuroanatomy of bipolar affective disorder: a critical review. Bipolar Disord 2001; 3: 106–50.

23. Strakowski SM, DelBello MP, Zimmerman ME, et al. Ventricular and periventricular structural volumes in first-versus multiple-episode bipolar disorder. Am J Psychiatry 2002; 159: 1841–7.

24. Escalona PR, Early B, McDonald WM, et al. Reduction of cerebellar volume in major depression: a controlled MRI study. Depression 1993; 1: 156–8.

25. Shah SA, Doraiswamy PM, Husain MM, et al. Posterior fossa abnormalities in major depression: a controlled magnetic resonance imaging study. Acta Psychiatr Scand 1992; 85: 474–79.

26. Swayze VW, Andreasen NC, Alligger RJ, et al. Subcortical and temporal structures in affective disorder and schizophrenia: a magnetic resonance imaging study. Biol Psychiatry 1992; 31: 221–40.

27. Harvey I, Persaud R, Ron MA, et al. Volumetric MRI measurements in bipolars compared with schizophrenics and healthy controls. Psychol Med 1994; 24: 689–99.

28. Strakowski SM, Wilson DR, Tohen M, et al. Structural brain abnormalities in first-episode mania. Biol Psychiatry 1993; 33: 602–9.

29. Dupont RM, Jernigan TL, Heindel W, et al. Magnetic resonance imaging and mood disorders. Localization of white matter and other subcortical abnormalities. Arch Gen Psychiatry 1995; 52: 747–55.

30. Strakowski SM, Adler CM, DelBello MP. Volumetric MRI studies of mood disorders: do they distinguish unipolar and bipolar disorders? Bipolar Disorders 2002; 4: 80–8.

31. Ongur D, Drevets WC, Price JL. Glial reduction in the subgenual prefrontal cortex in mood disorders. Proc Natl Acad Sci USA 1998; 95; 13290–5.

32. Videbech P. PET measurements of brain glucose metabolism and blood flow in major depressive disorder: a critical review. Acta Psychiatr Scand 2000; 101: 11–20.

33. Oquendo MA, Mann JJ. Serotonergic dysfunction in mood disorders. In Soares JC, Gershon S, eds. Bipolar Disorders: Basic Mechanisms and Therapeutic Implications. New York: Marcel Dekker, 2000: 121–42.

34. Baxter LR, Phelps ME, Mazziotta JC, et al. Cerebral metabolic rates for glucose in mood disorders: studies with positron emission tomography and fluorodeoxyglucose F18. Arch Gen Psychiatry 1985; 42: 441–7.

35. Cohen RM, Semple WE, Gross M, et al. Evidence for common alterations in cerebral glucose metabolism in major affective disorders and schizophrenia. Neuropsychopharmacology 1989; 2: 241–54.

36. al-Mousawi AH, Evans N, Ebmeier KP, et al. Limbic dysfunction in schizophrenia and mania. A study using ^{18}F-labelled fluorodeoxyglucose and positron emission tomography. Br J Psychiatry 1996; 169: 509–16.

37. Strakowski SM, DelBello MP, Adler CM, et al. Neuroimaging in bipolar disorder. Bipolar Disord 2000; 2: 148–64.

38. Blumberg HP, Stern E, Ricketts S, et al. Rostral and orbital prefrontal cortex dysfunction in manic state of bipolar disorder. Am J Psychiatry 1999; 156: 1986–8.

39. Ketter TA, Drevets WC. Neuroimaging studies of bipolar depression: functional neuropathology, treatment effects, and predictors of clinical response. Clin Neurosci Res 2002; 2: 182–92.

40. Blumberg HP, Leung H-C, Skundlarski P, et al. A functional magnetic resonance imaging study of bipolar disorder. Arch Gen Psychiatry 2003; 60: 601–9.

41. Rubinsztein JS, Fletcher PC, Rogers RD, et al. Decision-making in mania: a PET study. Brain 2001; 124: 2550–63.

42. Curtis VA, Dixon TA, Morris RG, et al. Differential activation in schizophrenia and bipolar illness during verbal fluency. J Affect Disord 2001; 66: 111–21.

43. Yurgelun-Todd DA, Gruber SA, Kanayama G, et al. fMRI during affect discrimination in bipolar affective disorder. Bipolar Disord 2000; 2: 237–48.

44. Baxter LR, Schwartz JM, Phelps ME, et al. Reduction of prefrontal cortex glucose metabolism common to three types of depression. Arch Gen Psychiatry 1989; 46: 243–50.

45. Buchsbaum MS, Wu J, DeLisi LE, et al. Frontal cortex and basal ganglia metabolic rates assessed by positron emission tomography with [^{18}F]2-deoxyglucose in affective illness. J Affect Disord 1986; 10: 137–52.

46. Morice R. Cognitive inflexibility and pre-frontal dysfunction in schizophrenia and mania. Br J Psychiatry 1990; 157: 50–4.

47. Hoff AL, Shukla S, Aronson T, et al. Failure to differentiate bipolar disorder from schizophrenia on measures of neuropsychological function. Schizophrenia Res 1990; 3: 253–60.

48. Hawkins KA, Hoffman RE, Quinlan DM, et al. Cognition, negative symptoms, and diagnosis: a comparison of schizophrenic, bipolar, and control samples. J Neuropsychiatry Clin Neurosci 1997; 9: 81–9.

49. Zihl J, Gron G, Brunnauer A. Cognitive deficits in schizophrenia and affective disorders: evidence for a final common pathway disorder. Acta Psychiatr Scand 1998; 97: 351–7.

50. Mayberg HS, Mahurin RK, Brannan SK. Neuropsychiatric aspects of mood and affective disorders. In Yudofsky SC, Hales RE, eds. The American Psychiatric Press Textbook of Neuropsychiatry, 3rd edn. Washington, DC: American Psychiatric Press, 1997: 883–902.

51. Bunney WEJ, Davis JM. Norepinephrine in depressive reactions. Arch Gen Psychiatry 1965, 13: 438–93.

52. Stefan M, Travis M, Murray RM. An Atlas of Schizophrenia. London: Parthenon Publishing, 2002.

53. Baldwin DS, Birtwhistle J. An Atlas of Depression. London: Parthenon Publishing, 2002.

54. Stahl SM. Essential Psychopharmacology of Depression and Bipolar Disorder. Cambridge: Cambridge University Press, 2000.

55. Pearlson GD, Wong DF, Tune LE, et al. In vivo D2 dopamine receptor density in psychotic and nonpsychotic patients with bipolar disorder. Arch Gen Psychiatry 1995, 52: 471–7.

56. Mann JJ, Arango V. Abnormalities of brain structure and function in mood disorders based on post-mortem investigations. In Charney DS, Nestler EJ, eds. Neurobiology of Mental Illness, 2nd edn. Oxford: Oxford University Press, 2004: 512–24.

57. Lorbcrboym M, Watemberg N, Nissenkorn A, et al. Technetium 99m ethylcysteinate dimer single emission computed tomography (SPECT) during intellectual stress test in children and adolescents with pure versus comorbid attention-deficit hyperactivity disorder (ADHD). J Child Neurol 2004, 19: 91–7.

5   Suicide and Bipolar Disorders: A Case Study

SUICIDE

Mood disorders have the power to kill. Far more than violence to others, individuals with bipolar disorders and unipolar depression are in danger of taking their own life. Goodwin and Jamison reviewed the research literature and reported that between 25 and 50% of people with bipolar disorders make a suicidal attempt at some point in their life (Figure 5.1)[1].

However, as Torrey and Knable point out, when one controls for studies that combined patients with bipolar and unipolar depression and those conducted before lithium was widely used, the incidence of attempted suicides is closer to 25%[2]. Estimates of completed suicides range from a low of 6 to 60%. When more specific definitions are used, and questionable studies are not included, it appears that the lifetime rate of completed suicides for bipolar patients is about 10% (Figure 5.2)[2].

There are only a few factors that differ between unipolar and bipolar completed suicides. Just before attempting suicide, unipolar patients may show more anxiety, agitation, and aggression than do people with bipolar disorder who are contemplating suicide. Bipolar II patients have higher rates of attempted and completed suicides than those with a bipolar I diagnosis. There is also evidence that people with bipolar illness who suffer from mixed episodes and delusional states are at an increased risk for suicide.

Women who have bipolar disorder follow the national trend for all categories of suicide and make more attempts. However, unlike the case of national suicide rates, men and women with bipolar disorders are almost even in terms of completed suicides[1].

Goodwin and Jamison report that, in a study of 54 adolescents who died from suicide, four factors accounted for 82% of the deaths[1,3]. Twenty-two percent of the sample had bipolar disorders, and about 11% had a diagnosis of unipolar depression.

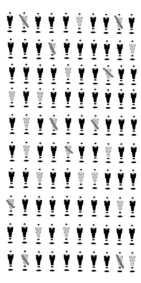

Figure 5.1 Suicide attempts and bipolar disorders. Twenty-five percent of people with bipolar illness will make at least one serious attempt to take their own life

---

Mixed episodes and rapid cycling increase the risk for suicide.

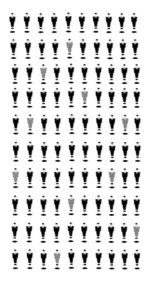

Figure 5.2 Bipolar disorders and deaths by suicide. Ten percent of people with bipolar illness will end their lives by committing suicide

Having bipolar illness accounted for more of the variance or predictive power compared with the other four factors.

Almost all studies find that having a bipolar disorder and abusing alcohol or other substances increases the risk of suicide and violence toward others, across the age spectrum. Torrey and Knable[2] found support in the literature for including the following eight items in suicidal assessments of patients with bipolar disorders:

(1) Family history of suicide, with risk increasing with seriousness of family attempts;

(2) Increased risk-taking or impulsiveness;

(3) Alcohol and substance abuse comorbid with bipolar disorder;

(4) Severity of clinical symptoms with particular attention to hopelessness, sleep disturbance, anxiety, and agitation;

(5) Increased isolation and/or no-one dependent or interpersonally close to the patient;

(6) Recent or increased life stressor;

(7) Poor response to psychotropic medications, or refusal to take medications;

(8) Time of year: in the past more suicides occurred in spring; however, newer data from England indicate that seasonal occurrences may no longer be as important.

The most robust indicators of suicide continue to be whether the patient has made a previous suicide attempt and has bipolar illness[1,4].

In addition to counting risk factors we also need to understand what the findings mean. Whether a patient's suicide risk is calculated through interviews and observations or suicide self-rating scales, the assigned score does not predict *per se* that the person will or will not make a suicide attempt. Identifying a higher number of indicators through an interview or the use of a rating scale places the patient in a group that has a higher probability for making a suicide attempt compared with someone with fewer risk factors. It is impossible, however, to predict who will actually try to take his or her life. We know that there will be people in the high-probability group who never make an attempt on their lives, and people in the low-probability group who will kill themselves. Additionally, not all risk items are weighted equally. As an example, having made previous attempts, using substances, and having access to weapons appear to have more predictive power than numerous other factors[1,2,4].

The preponderance of evidence overwhelmingly demonstrates that bipolar illness is a risk factor for suicide. Therefore, the importance for routinely assessing patients with any major mood disorder for suicidal thoughts and plans cannot be understated. It is also critical for family members to know how to identify suicidal thoughts and behaviors, and what to do when they occur. Many families need permission, reassurance, or concrete directions before feeling free to use hospital emergency rooms, telephone police, or use other crisis-workers for help. Their concerns, among other things, are that they may be mistaken and the person is not really suicidal, or that the ill member will refuse help and bolt. Families need to be reassured that they do not appear silly or incompetent, nor are they wasting the professional person's time when their suspicions of suicide are not validated by a mental health assessment.

VIOLENCE TO OTHERS

Mania has the ability to trigger verbal and physical aggression, while depression more often causes hypersensitivity, agitation, extreme pessimism and mild paranoia[1,4,5]. Shifts into any of these states can increase anxiety, reduce information-processing skills, and stir anger or defensive postures. Most often, the resulting aggression is in the form of verbal abuse, aggressive posturing, sudden anger, and abruptly leaving the setting. Mania, more than depression, can result in angry outbursts of unexpected physical aggression. The risk for behaviors such as pushing, fighting, destroying property, and driving in a rage increases as mania escalates. Physical acts also often quickly dissolve, resulting in little damage, but any violent behavior has potential for causing major injuries, financial and property losses, and legal ramifications. Severe depression, mania, and psychotic states result in far more suicides, self-mutilations, and minor to moderate property damage than homicide. Nonetheless, while it is rare, both bipolar depression and mania, particularly in combination with psychosis, can end in murder and manslaughter.

When a person is depressed, suicidal, or physically threatening to others but has no history of mania, there is a temptation quickly to prescribe or increase selective serotonin reuptake inhibitor (SSRI) medications. Generally, these drugs are known to reduce aggressive behaviors. Unfortunately, they also may increase suicidal thoughts in adolescents, and trigger severe manic episodes in patients with bipolar disorders, across the age spectrum[6]. If depression and aggressive behaviors or thoughts are increasing, and little is known about the patient's history, immediate hospitalization may be needed before antidepressants are introduced. This is particularly true if a patient has no history of

mania, but meets the criteria for a 'hidden' unexpressed bipolar disorder (see Chapter 6 for criteria).

POSTPARTUM DEPRESSION, PSYCHOSIS, AND BIPOLAR DISORDERS

Depression and psychosis can occur in mothers who have no history of mood disorders. However, the probability of developing postpartum depression or postpartum psychosis increases if the mother has previously had bipolar disorder, major depressive episodes, schizoaffective disorder, or postpartum depression/psychosis with the birth of any child. Having had postpartum depression with any previous birth increases the probability for it recurring with each future birth[7]. Pregnant women with a history of any psychiatric disorder, along with their partners and extended family members, may benefit from training that is more intense than that provided for mothers who are at less risk. These women should be screened several times during the first year after giving birth by a mental health expert knowledgeable of postpartum depression. All mothers and adult family members at a minimum require pre- and post-delivery training in how to recognize depression indicators, and differentiate between the 'baby blues' and postpartum depression.

The baby blues is not postpartum depression, but rather a combination of mild to severe physical, emotional, and cognitive symptoms experienced by as many as 50%[8] to 85%[7] of all new mothers. Because of the physical stress and sudden hormonal changes occurring immediately after birth it is common for mothers to acknowledge having the baby blues. Even women who have delivered other children may report that, either unlike or like in other births, they are experiencing emotional problems that range from mild to moderate in severity. Symptoms associated with the baby blues generally last for about the first 10 days after delivery, but may continue for several weeks.

Many women report that the severity of the symptoms peaked after the first week of delivery, and spontaneously disappeared during the second week[7]. Patients and families are advised to seek a professional psychiatric evaluation immediately if these or other signs of depression persist beyond 2 or 3 weeks.

Symptoms of Baby Blues

- Occur almost immediately after giving birth.
- Do not occur with every birth.
- Having not had the baby blues with a previous delivery does not signal that the symptoms will not appear when giving birth in the future.
- Having symptoms with one delivery does not predict that baby blues symptoms will appear in future births.
- Baby blues last between a few days and a few weeks, and spontaneously disappear.
- Major psychiatric symptoms include:
  - Fatigue;
  - Anxiety;
  - Irritability;
  - Crying (often for reasons the mother cannot explain);
  - Worry over mothering skills, ability to balance home, child care, work, and relationship responsibilities;
  - Inability to fall asleep;
  - Appetite fluctuations and sudden weight gain and loss.

POSTPARTUM DEPRESSION

Unlike the baby blues, postpartum depression will last longer than a few days or weeks, may appear at any time during the child's first year of life, often causes more severe symptoms, and is less likely simply to disappear with time. Researchers currently debate whether postpartum depression can occur beyond the child's first birthday. People are surprised to discover that this is not a rare psychiatric disorder. Approximately one in ten and up to 15% of women having a baby experience mild to severe postpartum depression[7,9]. The large number of postpartum episodes occurs at least in part because a number of women deliver children having an undiagnosed and untreated depression or bipolar disorder. One study using self-report rating scales with 3472 pregnant women found that 20% scored above the clinical cut-off score for depression. That is, the screening instrument found that approximately 694 women warranted a full assessment for depression. Furthermore, only 14% of those identified as possibly having depression were receiving treatment[10]. Hidden disorders place mothers at greater risk for postpartum depression, and prevent medical providers from assertively providing preventive treatments and support. Additionally, women who unknowingly suffer from mild bipolar II disorder or cyclothymia are at added risk for having their depression symptoms misdiagnosed and treated with only an antidepressant.

It is important for families to understand that postpartum depression is more than simply feeling sad, worried, or anxious. Without coaching and education, family members and friends may disregard and even refuse to listen to a mother's ruminations about not being able to care for the baby or to provide adequate attention and love. Culture teaches that women biologically and emotionally are made to have and care for a baby. Families and community leaders literally do not know how to respond to a mother's expressions of doubt or fear. They often view the mother's concerns as overstatements, drama, or fatigue that will quickly pass. It is extremely difficult for a mother who is developing postpartum depression to be heard and validated by her support systems. Without guidance, families find it impossible to comprehend how a mother who, before giving birth, looked joyfully forward to parenting, is now painfully and completely convinced that she cannot today, tomorrow, or ever rise to the occasion of nurturing, protecting, and physically caring for a child. Even more baffling for people is why the mother is not consoled by concrete help and reassurance, and why she simply does not 'function' regardless of her self-perceptions and feelings. It is extremely difficult for untrained individuals to independently grasp that depression removes one's ability to cognitively and emotionally discover or accept alternative solutions. For an untrained person who has never been depressed it is difficult to understand that the patient is not simply rejecting advice, but is unable to perceive that unexplored solutions and hope realistically exist. Additionally, mothers and family members are reluctant to initiate a discussion about depression with their internal medicine doctor, let alone mental health professionals. As a result, health and mental health providers have to be assertive, yet sensitive to the fact that a mother's ambivalence may stem from:

(1) Lack of awareness and understanding about what is happening to her;

(2) Cultural beliefs, or significant family members and supporting community who do not believe in psychotropic medications, and define depression as a choice or character flaw;

(3) Self-shame, embarrassment, and guilt;

(4) Fear that she will be reported to child-protection services and her baby will be placed in a foster home;

(5) Belief that her family and friends will not understand;

(6) Lack of awareness that treatments are effective, and one does not have to 'tough it out';

(7) Loss of energy and ability to plan cognitively how to obtain help.

Perhaps one of the most common symptoms seen in postpartum depression is obsessive thoughts randomly occurring throughout each day[7,11]. The thoughts usually focus on a central theme such as lacking ability to care for the child, unworthiness to be a mother, inability to protect the child from lurking worldly dangers, fear and belief that the baby is in pain, or physical problems causing personal fatigue. Research indicates that self-criticism makes a new mother more vulnerable to postpartum depression[11]. In addition to obsessive themes, any of the symptoms below that repetitively appear, disappear, and then return, or are observed on most days for an extended period, may indicate postpartum depression[7,8]:

(1) Doubting abilities to mother and care for the child's welfare;

(2) Recurring fear or anxiety that she is going to injure the baby;

(3) Obsessive worries (which may focus on issues other than the baby, such as finances, religious beliefs, or current world affairs);

(4) Having little or no interest in the baby (for example, holding the baby may provide no internal reward);

(5) Feeling overly upset when the baby cannot be satisfied or will not sleep;

(6) Crying for no known reason at random times, or not able to cry (she may state that she feels too numb to cry, or is unable to identify why crying does not occur);

(7) Sleeping too little or too much (a general pattern is waking after having been asleep and being unable to get back to sleep);

(8) Difficulty in making decisions;

(9) Changes in eating habits;

(10) Self-blame;

(11) Nothing is seen as humorous or funny;

(12) Irritability or anger that is more intense than the triggering event, or occurs for no known reason;

(13) Ongoing or recurring guilt (she may feel guilty for brining the child into the world);

(14) Loss of enjoyment in things that were previously rewarding or satisfying

(15) Inability to relax;

(16) Feeling empty;

(17) Chronic physical problems (e.g. pain, digestive problems, headaches);

(18) Skills for functioning in social situations, work settings, or school have significantly decreased;

(19) Thoughts of hopelessness or pessimism;

(20) Thoughts of death, suicide, or homicide.

POSTPARTUM PSYCHOSIS

A small number of mothers experiencing postpartum depression will continue a downward course and spiral into an episode of postpartum psychosis. This occurs in approximately 1 per 1000 births[8]. Disordered thinking, loss of reality, reduced ability for abstract thinking, and increased negative symptoms may be more prominent than obvious hallucinations and delusions. Patients who have a history of bipolar disorder can move into psychosis from either a depressive or a manic episode. In the midst of a psychotic episode the person's altered reality can override solidly developed moral codes and usher in tragic behaviors that leave scarred memories throughout the family and even the community. The following is an example of how untreated postpartum depression evolved into postpartum psychosis, and in the shortest of time resulted in an unpredicted and unthinkable tragedy.

THE STORY OF MINE*

She was brilliant, on the very edge of making a mark in academia, until postpartum depression ushered in pain, confusion, and the horror of two unexpected deaths. Mine was fluent in English, French, Turkish, and several Arabic dialects. Both before and after receiving her doctorate, Mine traveled throughout the Middle East and Europe developing research studies and speaking in the defense of the poorest of the poor. In Cairo and Istanbul her efforts helped to increase awareness of government-sponsored assistance for the destitute. With knowledge and compassion, Mine had the ability to change how people and governments understood the responsibility, purpose, and role of charity. Colleagues credit Mine as one of those rare individuals who could comprehend all of the dimensions of an issue, and yet embrace criticism. Her energy and dedication seemed boundless. Mine's final book, *Managing Egypt's Poor and the Politics of Benevolence, 1800–1952*, published by Princeton University Press in 2003, used police and other historical records to interpret the historical interplay between philanthropy, politics, and the poor. She was determined to create change and promote social justice by giving a voice and history to forgotten beggars, and families drowning in, yet surviving in, hopeless poverty (Figure 5.3).

As Mine turned 38 years old, she was a successful academic, happily married, in good health with no history of mental illness, excited about being pregnant, and eternally optimistic. She was contagiously happy, and people gravitated to her. Sadly, in the fall of 2003, shortly after the birth of a child with Down's syndrome, Mine was swallowed up by the overwhelming despair of postpartum depression.

*The author wishes to thank Mine's family for sharing this important story and allowing it to be published.

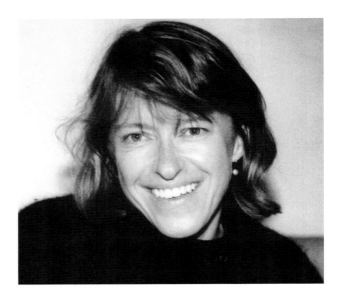

Figure 5.3 Mine before the onset of postpartum depression and psychosis. She was energetic, happy, and successful

From joy to depression and psychosis

The news that her baby, named Raya, had Down's syndrome was met with determination, acceptance, and appropriate concern. True to her nature, Mine dove into books on caring for a Down's syndrome baby, organizing notes, developing resource files, and 'case-managing' a host of specialist and community agencies. Not atypical for Down's syndrome babies, Raya was unable to develop a strong enough sucking response for breast- or bottle-feeding. To resolve the problem, a nasal/gastric feeding tube was inserted. This added work and difficulty for Mine and her husband, but did not deter their optimism, energy, and parental dedication. For the first 4 months, Mine was a determined mother providing emotional and physical care. Family members marveled at how smoothly she managed the added work created by the feeding tube and other care requirements. In these early months, Mine was forever holding, rocking, and talking to Raya (Figure 5.4).

The baby's smile delighted both Mine and her husband. In addition, she told friends and family that Raya slept well, seldom fussed, and was amazingly accommodating. The family saw a woman successfully balancing a spousal relationship, professional obligations, and motherhood.

During a visit to her family in Saint Paul, Minnesota, hints of a problem and change in Mine became apparent for the first time as the baby

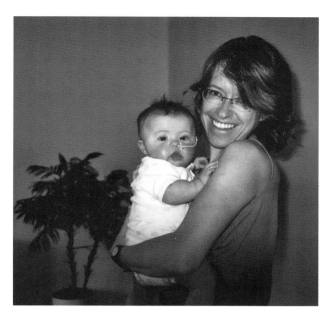

Figure 5.4 Mine and Raya, June 2003. A relaxed Mine and baby without obvious signs of postpartum depression. People can often hide symptoms, continue with life, and pretend that things will get better when depression first starts

turned 5 months old. She became quieter, needed more rest, and expressed concerns for the baby. Mine was also starting to express worries that the baby was not eating enough and would have to continue using a feeding tube. The family recalls that while it would be unfair to say that she obsessed about the child's nutrition, it clearly had become a focus of her attention and a repeated theme. Yet, in the eyes of friends and family, Mine continued to appear happy, calm, and in control of herself and the baby. Pictures taken during this period show a mother and baby spontaneously smiling at each other. One month later Mine cut short a vacation, and went to her mother's house in Saint Paul, where she had grown up.

Upon arrival she was visibly depressed, upset, and physically stressed. Mine's voice was weak, her body held in an uncomfortable tense posture. Sorrow and despair were reflected in her face. Most of the coping skills she was known for were gone. In a defeated tone, Mine told how she could no longer care for Raya, that it was too difficult. The family rallied around her, and intuitively knew not to leave Mine alone. Within days, as the list of symptoms increased, the family grew painfully aware that professional help was needed. Sadness, anger, and anxiety filled Mine's face most of each day. Feeding the baby had

become an odious and difficult task. When nursing, Mine held her upper body in a tense fashion and anxiously pushed up on the balls of her feet. She was obsessed with the idea that her breast-milk lacked any nutrition. Mine saw her milk as having the consistency of water, even though, when refrigerated, cream formed at the top. At some feedings the breast-milk was discarded or fortified with formula powder out of fear that it was only water. Throughout the week, Mine obsessively complained that Raya was not getting enough food. Attempts to reassure her that the baby appeared healthy and was gaining weight were met with silence or partially stated arguments. Mine hardly ate, stating that she could no longer taste food. Instead of sleeping, nights were spent awake worrying about Raya. Between feedings, Mine was often agitated; she paced, momentarily lay on a couch in a semi-fetal position, then resumed pacing. She often made sounds of crying, but produced no tears. Most mornings Mine ruminated over and over that she could no longer care for Raya. Evenings were better. Mine became more composed, less upset, and able to make business calls and engage with the family in light conversation.

After 2 days, the family searched for resources, and a psychologist known for working with mothers and postpartum depression was recommended. After another day passed, contact was made with the psychologist and an appointment made for the following day. Mine agreed to go, but insisted that no one could help. She told the family that all of this was her fault. Earlier, Mine had told the family that in addition to not getting enough to eat, the baby was completely deaf, and shook or trembled. The family observed signs of the baby responding to sounds, and never witnessed any spasms. Mine's sister-in-law took her for the appointment with the psychologist. Mine decided to go into the session alone, without her sister-in-law. On the drive home, Mine showed her sister-in-law a list of emergency numbers provided by the psychologist, and volunteered that the meeting was not very helpful.

The following morning Mine's symptoms escalated. At one point she looked at her mother and said, 'Mom, I'm sorry if something worse should happen.' Her worry that Raya was only getting water from the breast-milk was also intensifying. Mine told her sister-in-law that she did not want help, that it would not change the fact that Raya was sick and had no future. Additionally, for the first time, Mine stated openly that she wanted to die. This prompted another call and visit to the psychologist. The meeting produced a recommendation to see a doctor immediately who could prescribe medication therapy. After much telephoning, and repeating their story to receptionists, a family doctor gave Mine a late-afternoon appointment. The doctor invited a family member to remain for the meeting, and Mine did not object. Mine answered the assessment questions in a surprisingly forthright manner. Among other things, she told the doctor about having thoughts of jumping into the Mississippi River, and her concerns of not being able to care for Raya. Mine was prescribed Celexa® (citalopram) and sent home.

The next day, Saturday, Mine obsessed over and over about her fear that the baby was starving. She would let out long breaths of air in a forced sighing manner, and declare that because of her, the baby's life was shattered and doomed. A call expressing concern over Mine's obsessing and increased negative statements was placed to the psychologist. The family was encouraged to have Mine see the psychiatrist on Monday. Throughout the remaining part of the weekend someone from the family was with Mine. On Sunday she was still agitated, but able to participate in a small birthday party for her mother. At one point she became cross with her brother, but seemed less obsessed and irritated than had been observed on Saturday. The family closed out the weekend worried, but hopeful that the medication would start making things better, determined to have Mine see the psychiatrist Monday, and very tired.

On Monday morning just after 9:00 a.m., after finishing the morning feeding, Mine walked with Raya to the bathroom and cut the baby's throat twice with a kitchen knife. Mine then walked back to the kitchen without Raya and told her mother in a flat, monotone voice without emotion, 'I just killed my baby' (Figure 5.5). The paramedics were called, and they subsequently called the police. Mine was taken to the county jail and charged with murder. Her lawyer's request for hospitalization was turned down. Bail was set at $500 000. Psychiatric assessments by the forensic psychiatrist revealed that Mine's postpartum depression had spiraled into psychosis. For about a month prior to killing Raya, Mine had had delusions, and auditory and visual hallucinations.

Mine was placed on an antipsychotic and antidepressant medication, but was not put on a formal suicide watch despite repeated requests by family

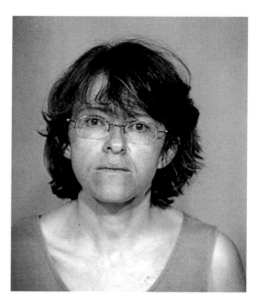

Figure 5.5 Mine in a tense state of depression and psychosis (August 4, 2003). This police photo shows how depression and psychosis stresses, confuses, and changes the very physical features of a person

members to police, detention-center guards, nurses, and deputies. County jail authorities simply assured the family that Mine would be closely observed (Figures 5.6–5.9). Two weeks later she was discovered making a noose out of sheets, and given a tighter watch order. However, Mine was not seen by a psychiatrist for 3 days after being found preparing to kill herself. To help prevent suicide, she was dressed in a rip-proof Kevlar® gown that was supposed to fasten with Velcro®. Unfortunately, the strips were so worn that the gown would not remain closed. When around people, she had to hold the gown closed. The gown, without repair, was also worn and covered with a blanket during Mine's second public court hearing. Requests for hospitalization were constantly made by the family and rejected by the authorities.

Within days of the last request for hospital care and the previous suicide attempt, Mine would end her ordeal. In a 24-hour lighted concrete-walled observation dormitory under a blanket, Mine covered her head with a plastic garbage bag stolen earlier in the day, pulled it tightly to ensure that no air could enter, and alone on a floor mat suffocated to death.

Since Mine's death, a postscript is required. Because of her contributions to the university where she worked as a 'scholar, teacher, mentor, friend', her university department dedicated a memorial plaque

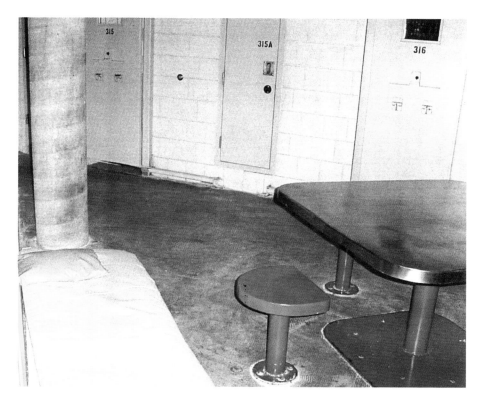

Figure 5.6 Day-room where Mine was imprisoned under suicide watch. Mine was not in a jail cell, but rather on a mat in the common day-room. Next to her mat that served as a bed was glass that allowed correctional officers to observe her actions. However, because of the constant bright lights, inmates often covered their heads with blankets. Mine's blanket was used to hide her suicidal death

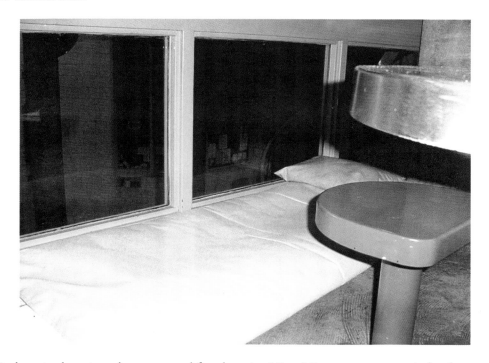

Figure 5.7 Windows in the prison day-room used for observing Mine. Mine serves as a reminder that casual and distant observation alone will not keep a severely depressed person safe from suicide. The cold and stark prison atmosphere at best does not help mentally ill individuals, and may interact with their brain disorder, causing increased depression, mania, or psychosis

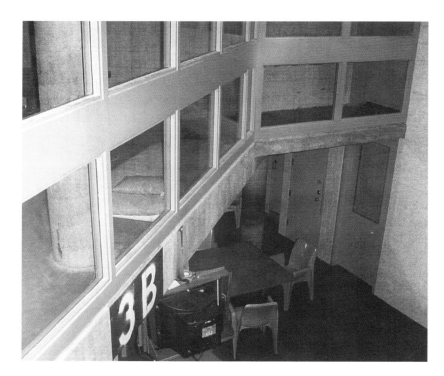

Figure 5.8 Observing Mine. Mine's sleeping area above the day-room documents that an attempt was made to observe her behaviors. Unfortunately, arrangements of this type place the prisoner at a distance from the security personnel. Additionally, the window frames and certain viewing angles can obscure what the person is or is not doing. As Mine proved, observation rooms of this type make small hidden movements and behaviors difficult for even trained security personnel to detect. Mentally ill people who are suicidal need to be hospitalized and monitored on a one-to-one basis.

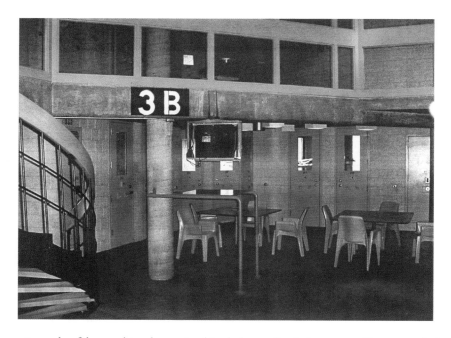

Figure 5.9 Mine spent much of her waking hours in this drab, confined day-room. She entered the prison depressed, confused, psychotic, and unable to stop her obsessional thoughts. Living in an environment with little visual stimulation, minimum contact with known, trusted people, and 24-hour lighting can increase these symptoms, reinforce feelings of hopelessness, and accelerate suicidal behaviors. While the day-room and sleeping areas are relatively small, they are nonetheless large enough to allow individual behaviors to go unobserved. Mine's sleeping pad, next to the window with a sheet of paper, can barely be seen in this photo

in her honor. The tribute was viewed by a significant number of people on and off campus as being inappropriate, and was met by a demand for the plaque to be removed. The protestors were neither willing to honor the good Mine had done for others, nor listen to scientific facts of how her actions arose from a neurobiological illness, and not from selfishness, corrupted values, or wickedness.

Lessons from a tragedy

Mine had classic symptoms of postpartum depression, hints of psychosis, and concrete suicidal warning signs. Yet, two professionals failed to suggest, let alone push for, hospitalization. While homicidal thoughts were never expressed, her beliefs that the baby was suffering, dying slowly from starvation, and that she was helpless to save the child, were communicated over and over. Messages given this strongly and persistently signal the need for in-patient care. The signal may have been missed because a complete interview and assessment were not done with both the patient and her family.

In such a case, a thorough diagnostic interview with the family would have revealed information suggesting that Mine's depression had turned into a psychosis. The patient's inability to accept, even when shown, that her milk contained cream, and incorrectly perceiving the baby as having spasms, hint at the possibility of her having been delusional. Even had suicidal or delusional thoughts not been present, a short in-patient stay deserved consideration. The patient's social and work skills had substantially decreased, she obsessed in a manner that hinted that psychosis might be present, and she perceived herself as causing the baby's problems. Her state of mind was unpredictable, and was showing no sign of improving. Furthermore, because of the level of severity and complications, medication decisions needed careful consideration and assessment.

Use of a multidisciplinary psychiatric team in this situation would have provided neuropsychological assessments, genetic histories, social–environmental assessments, and in-depth interviews with the family. These tools would have greatly assisted the psychiatrist in making medication decisions and treatment plans. This case did not get to a multidisciplinary psychiatric team in part because the family was not encouraged to take Mine immediately to a hospital emergency room. There is a need for public service announcements that teach how to recognize psychi-

atric emergencies, and when to take a person directly to an emergency room.

This case also illustrates how the severity of depression can be missed when families are not included in the assessment process. The psychologist followed the patient's wishes without protest and excluded her sister-in-law. The general practitioner included the family, but directed the assessment to the patient. That is, the family was more in an observer role, and used primarily when clarifications were needed. In assessing any form of severe depression or mania, family members need to be full participants. Additionally, although there was mention of an increased suicide risk and a need to be watchful, neither of the professionals provided a complete plan to the patient and family for preventing suicide, and no follow-up appointments were initiated. Mine planned to return to Philadelphia within a week. Nonetheless, considering her symptom severity, an in-office appointment along with scheduled phone support conferences should have been strongly recommended by the psychologist and medical doctor. It is also important to note that the doctor assumed that Mine had postpartum depression. No attempt was made to determine whether there were indicators of undiagnosed hypomanic episodes, or a family history of bipolar disorder or mania. Under the circumstances, one could question whether Mine's high level of energy, work habits, and love of running suggested periods of hypomania.

Additionally, the Mine tragedy underscores at least three problems in caring for people suffering with a major mental disorder. Perhaps most important, it illustrates that mental health systems continue to have difficulty in preventing a life-threatening crisis, and in assuring that people can quickly gain access to a wide range of services. Neither Mine nor her family had been prepared to recognize postpartum depression and understand that hospitalization was critically needed. Furthermore, the family found it difficult to receive professional advice and support quickly. A family that had never seen severe mental illness was forced to make major decisions in a vacuum. Appropriate training about postpartum depression and immediate professional intervention would have led to a high probability of saving Mine and her baby. This tragedy illustrates that service delivery problems spelled out in the United States' Surgeon General's Report on Mental Illness are real and deadly.

Mine's experience with the law enforcement system also highlights how law and policies regulating the incarceration of mentally ill people have failed to keep up with modern scientific knowledge. Newer empirically documented knowledge about mental disorders is not being disseminated and integrated into public policies and budgets. Our legal systems, as an example, have yet to consider fully that mental illnesses are neurobiological in nature and change the very structure and functioning of the brain. Legal restrictions and outdated definitions of mental illness often prevent jurors from considering how depression, mania, and psychosis distort reality, remove choices, and shape behavior. A person with severe depression or mania may retrospectively understand that an act is legally wrong. This does not, however, address whether the person had the same understanding as the behavior was being performed. Policies have yet to reflect how scientific findings such as changes in the frontal cortex that alter judgment and problem-solving, or an overly functioning limbic system that floods the mind with emotions and distorted memories, apply in criminal and civil law. Additionally, federal and state sentencing rules, treatment accommodation, and care requirements for imprisoned mentally ill people seldom follow best-practice guidelines. There is a high probability that Mine's death would had been prevented had she been sent to a forensic psychiatric hospital, or placed on a one-to-one constant suicide watch in the county jail.

Finally, the fact that Mine's university was forced to remove a memorial plaque dedicated to the remembrance of her service, teaching, and research sadly illustrates that mental illness is not even understood within centers of education, much less by the general public. The student and faculty reaction underscores that the mentally ill continue to be stigmatized, incorrectly labeled, and placed out of the public's consciousness. It further helps to explain why mentally ill people hide their difficulties, and refuse to seek professional help until they are in the center of an uncontrollable crisis. Mine's family is overcoming their grief by advocating for:

(1) Continuing education requirements undertaken by mental-health professionals to include training in postpartum depression, and postpartum psychosis;

(2) Mothers and families to receive improved postpartum education, assessment, and support before and after the baby is born;

(3) Legislation requiring incarcerated mentally ill people to receive improved living conditions, assessments, therapy, and suicide prevention.

The family sincerely hopes that out of the darkness of grief and tragedy, positive change will occur. Largely because of their efforts, the county jail where Mine died has promised significant revisions of their policies and methods for protecting prisoners at risk for suicide.

AN OUTLINE FOR PREVENTING TRAGEDY

A planned program can prevent postpartum depression and postpartum psychosis from escalating into irreversible tragedy. A comprehensive program starts during the mother's pregnancy and continues after the child is born. The proposed recommendations include services to mothers and their families in both the pre-delivery and post-delivery periods. Culturally competent education, assessment, support, and treatment when needed can substantially reduce the risks of postpartum depression. While the outline is idealistic, the steps have been developed through interviews by the author with women and family members who have experienced the hardships of postpartum depression and the return of bipolar illness following delivery. Clinics and community organizations may want to consider altering and building on the broad steps outlined below.

Pre-delivery phase: prevention during pregnancy

(1) Mother, father, and extended adult family members require education about postpartum depression:

(a) What it is and why it is a biological illness;

(b) Why postpartum depression is not a sign of weakness or a character flaw;

(c) The importance and effectiveness of psychiatric treatment;

(d) How to identify onset or risk indicators;

(e) When and how to seek professional help.

(2) Every mother is screened at each trimester of pregnancy for depression using a brief semi-structured interview and self-rating scales.

(3) The mother's psychiatric history is gained using questionnaires and semi-structured interviews:

(a) The interview and questionnaire must be structured to identify all previously treated and untreated psychiatric disorders.

(b) Special attention and skill are needed for identifying untreated and previously undiagnosed dysthymia, cyclothymia, and hypomania.

(c) Mothers who may have had cyclothymia or hypomania should not be given an anti-depressant as a monotherapy (see Chapter 6).

(4) A genetic history for the mother's family is conducted using questionnaires and interviews:

(a) When possible, identify diagnosed mental disorders and indicators of undiagnosed disorders for the past two or more generations.

(b) Ask questions that help to identify undiagnosed addictions, alcohol abuse, all major mood disorders, schizoaffective disorder, major anxiety disorders, and psychosis across family members and generations.

Post-delivery phase: prevention after delivery

(1) A packet and video are to be sent home with the family after birth reminding them that the baby blues are normal, and explaining how to identify signs of depression, the importance of support, and how and when to obtain professional help.

(2) Depression screening is to be carried out by health professionals 3 weeks after the baby is delivered, and thereafter every 3–4 months during the first year.

(3) Mother and family education and consulting should be available upon request.

(4) Planned contact by mail, email, or phone provides support and gives family permission to discuss concerns.

(5) The mother is provided with depression self-rating scales and encouraged to track her mood and discuss ratings during phone conferences; she is encouraged to do self-ratings at weeks 3, 6, 8, and every 4–6 months thereafter for the first year.

The outline represents an idealized process that most clinics, because of limited resources, could not completely replicate. Medical insurance seldom covers this much personalized education, assessment, and follow-up. The steps nonetheless are presented to underscore two important points. First, education for postpartum depression, as for all disorders, must always include the family. Fathers, partners, and grandparents need to understand depression and know how and when to provide support. Furthermore, mothers in a state of depression cannot be expected to defy their family or culture and independently seek help. Strength and advocacy for using professional mental health resources must come from the family, not from within the mother. Finally, an idealized program is suggested to illustrate that prevention of postpartum depression and postpartum psychosis is possible, but will not materialize until a mandate, resources, and education are provided by governments, professional mental-health associations, businesses, and educational institutions.

Post-partum questionnaires are provided in Appendix 1.

REFERENCES

1. Goodwin FK, Jamison KR. Manic–Depressive Illness. New York: Oxford University Press, 1990.

2. Torrey EF, Knable MB. Surviving Manic Depression: A Manual on Bipolar Disorder for Patients, Families and Providers. New York: Basic Books, 2002.

3. Brent DA, Perper JA, Goldstein CE, et al. Risk factors for adolescent suicide: a comparison of adolescent suicide victims with suicidal inpatients. Arch Gen Psychiatry 1988; 45: 581–8.

4. Jamison KR. Night Falls Fast. New York: Vintage Books, 1999.

5. Geller B, DelBello MP, eds. Bipolar Disorder in Childhood and Early Adolescence. New York: Guilford Press, 2003.

6. Stahl SM. Essential Psychopharmacology of Depression and Bipolar Disorder. Cambridge: Cambridge University Press, 2000.

7. Burt VK, Hendrick VC. Women's mental health. In Hales RE, Yudofsky SC, eds. The American Psychiatric Publishing Textbook of Clinical Psychiatry, 4th edn. Washington, DC: American Psychiatric Publishing, 2003: 1511–33.

8. Sadock BJ, Sadock VA. Synopsis of Psychiatry Behavioral Sciences/Clinical Psychiatry, 9th edn. Philadelphia: Lippincott Williams & Wilkins, 2003.

9. Nolen-Hoeksema S. Gender differences in depression. In Gotlib IH, Hammen CL, eds. Handbook of Depression. New York: The Guilford Press, 2002: 492–509.

10. Marcus SM, Flynn HA, Blow FC, Barry K. Depressive symptoms among pregnant women screened in obstetrics settings. J Women's Health 2003, 12: 373–80.

11. Blatt SJ. Experiences of Depression: Theoretical, Clinical, and Research Perspectives. Washington, DC: American Psychological Association, 2004.

6   Treating Bipolar Disorders

Effective treatment for depression, mania, and mixed episodes triggered by bipolar I, bipolar II, and schizoaffective disorders requires professionally prescribed and supervised psychotropic medications. Rehabilitation starts when patients understand that symptoms are not psychological mirages hiding deep, tragic secrets or self-induced emotional injuries, but rather indicators of a serious and real illness that, without medications, will not improve. The primary treatment goal for all bipolar disorders is to end destructive symptoms and return patients to their normal level of functioning. In their classic textbook, Goodwin and Jamison stress the importance of patients receiving early, timely, and aggressive treat-ment for bipolar disorders[1]. Delaying treatment and hoping that symptoms will disappear as mysteriously as they arrived can end in disaster. Untreated depressive and manic episodes can increase illness severity, decrease the length of time between episodes, damage biological brain structures, and increase the risk of suicide (Figure 6.1)[1,2].

While medications are the first step toward rehabilitation, a comprehensive treatment plan also includes (Figure 6.2):

(1)   Medication education;

(2)   Education for patients, families, and significant others about bipolar disorders;

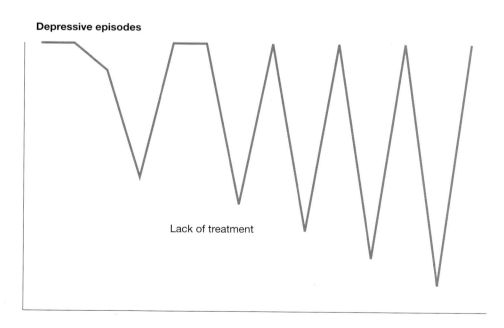

Figure 6.1   When left untreated, depressive episodes increase in duration and the time between episodes decreases

(3) Assistance in learning how to identify early warning signs, and the difference between normal mood changes and bipolar episodes;

(4) Appropriate psychotherapies;

(5) Support for both the patient and the family.

Each of these five treatment components is important; nonetheless, any treatment for bipolar disorders that does not immediately emphasize and place drug therapy as the central ingredient for overcoming symptoms must be seen as suspect and highly questionable by consumers.

No form of treatment currently known can cure bipolar disorders. As in diabetes, bipolar symptoms for many people can be muted and controlled, allowing individuals to live industrious, meaningful lives, but they are not cured and free from their brain disease. For most patients with bipolar I, II, or schizoaffective disorder, medication treatment will become a lifelong requirement. Therefore, education and technical information will periodically require updating. The need for and appropriateness of psychotherapy is largely dictated by a patient's personal and family problems, medication reactions, and environmental events. Because this is a long-term chronic illness, the amount of support required by a patient, family, or significant others waxes and wanes. Support needs change not only with the onset and severity of illness episodes but also from shifts or

changes in national and personal economics, transportation availability, housing costs or tenant rules, relationships, legal problems, work or school requirements, and numerous environmental settings and ecological systems that have uniquely met the person's emotional needs.

Today, treatment for bipolar disorders attempts not simply to react from crisis to crisis responding to manic or depressive episodes, but rather to treat the entire illness comprehensively and support the person's strengths throughout the life cycle and across the his or her environmental settings (Figure 6.3).

A person's illness can be helped by treating first the brain disorder and simultaneously influences coming from the patient's behavior, cognition, emotional responses, and environment. In addition to medication case-management, direct assertive advocacy is often required for medical interventions to succeed. Treatment will make no progress if patients lack funds for, access to, or understanding of medication. Cultural, economic, and legal factors must be attended to throughout the treatment process. The 'brain–environment' diagram emphasizes that the treatment progress can be undermined by numerous human, sociocultural, and even political interacting factors.

When acute episodes subside, treatment immediately shifts from focusing on an episodic crisis to

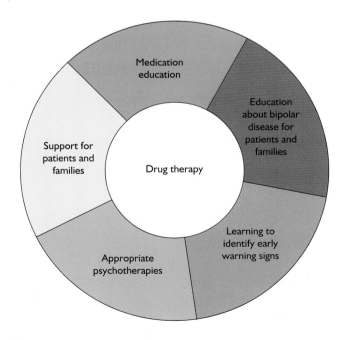

Figure 6.2 Comprehensive treatment

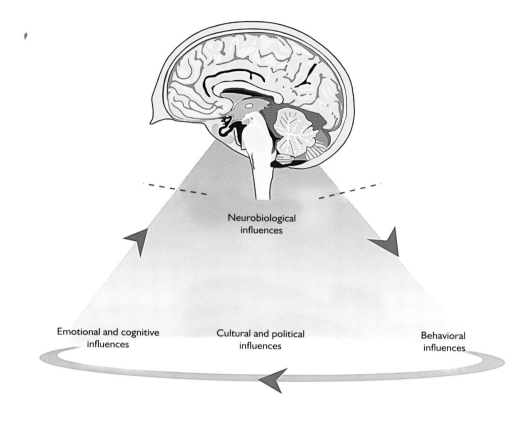

Figure 6.3 Brain–environment focus of treatment. This illustrates the interaction between biological and ecological factors. The brain must be treated first, but psychological, emotional, and political–cultural factors can help or block effective treatment. Additionally, the brain when in a manic or depressed state can stop positive factors from past learning, personal and interpersonal experiences, and society from being helpful. Ecological systems can block assistance to the brain, and our brain can block assistance from social systems and personal strengths

managing and improving persistent chronic minor symptoms, fears, and disabling habits that inhibit personal growth, and substantially increasing interpersonal relationships and quality of life[3]. Additionally, during periods when depression and mania are in remission, patients have time, energy, and the cognitive skills required to improve their personal talents and strengths. Maintenance therapy always includes medication adjustment and supervision, and often incorporates individualized psychotherapies and structured support for reinforcing and improving the person's strengths.

MEDICATIONS, THE FIRST LINE OF TREATMENT

A person's first-onset symptoms of a bipolar disorder can have the hallmarks of classical unipolar depres-

sion. This presents a dilemma for medical doctors. Imipramine and other tricyclic medications, widely used for depression and often less expensive than newer drugs, may induce mania. This is less true with monoamine oxidase inhibitor (MAOI) antidepressants (Table 6.1). These drugs, while safer, will push some patients into a severe manic episode. Additionally, patients find the highly restrictive food and beverage requirements, which absolutely must be followed while taking MAOI medications, extremely difficult to follow (Table 6.2).

Even the new generation of selective serotonin reuptake inhibitor (SSRI) drugs poses a danger for a person with bipolar depression[6]. SSRIs have become the treatment of choice for individuals with major unipolar depression. Their effectiveness, however, appears to be no better than that of the older tricyclic antidepressants. However, compared with tricyclics such as imipramine, SSRIs are safer, have

Table 6.1 Side-effects of monoamine oxidase inhibitor (MAOI) antidepressants: isocarboxazid (Marplan®), phenelzine (Nardil®), and tranylcypromine (Parnate®)

	Common	Uncommon
Allergies or rashes		✓
Blurred vision	✓	
Chest pain		✓
Chills or shivering		✓
Constipation or diarrhea		✓
Decreased sexual ability	✓	
Dizziness or light-headedness	✓	
Drowsiness or weakness	✓	
Dry mouth	✓	
Fast or slow heartbeat	✓	
Severe headache		✓
Weight gain	✓	

fewer side-effects, are better tolerated physically, and less often increase or induce manic symptoms[6]. Yet SSRIs are associated with triggering mania in up to 20% of people with a bipolar disorder[7].

Additionally, a condition known as serotonin syndrome can occur if SSRI medications cause an overabundance of serotonin to be released in the brain and peripheral nervous system. This is a rather rare reaction identified by symptoms that include headaches, diarrhea, chills, sweating, dizziness, agitation, confusion, excitation, disorientation, elevated temperatures, increased blood pressure, palpitations, restlessness, unsteady gait, increased muscle tone with twitching, tremor, myoclonic jerks, hyperreflexia, and delirium. While this is a rare reaction, it is extremely dangerous, and can result in coma and death. Patients taking multiple drugs acting on the brain's serotonin system are at a higher risk for developing the syndrome. The symptoms most often occur within 24 h of starting an SSRI, an overdose of the drug, or a change in the prescribed dosage. Several deaths have been presumed to be related to serotonin syndrome from a combination of SSRIs

Table 6.2 Monoamine oxidase inhibitor (MAOI) restriction list. Combined from references 4 and 5

Foods to avoid	Foods to use only in small limited amounts	Examples of drugs that interact with MAOIs (avoid with MAOIs)

Banana skins and over-ripe (aged) fruit
Beef and chicken livers
Brewer's yeast
Broad-bean pods
Canned figs
Fava beans
Fermented products (such as fermented or preserved fish, liver, and meats)
Monosodium glutamate
Pickled fish (e.g. pickled herring, sardines, and anchovies)
Red wine
Ripe cheeses (except cream-cheese)
Sauerkraut
Sausage, salami
Sherry, liqueurs
Yeast extracts
Yogurt and sour cream
	Caffeinated beverages and food, e.g.:
	  Chocolate
	  Coffee
	  Colas
	  Tea
	Soy sauce
	Beer
	Wines other than red wine
		Causes highly dangerous interaction:
		  MAOI switching (remain off MAOI at least 1 week before switching to new or different MAOI)
		  Meperidine (interaction could be fatal)
		  Dextromethorphan (interaction reported to cause brief psychosis)
		  Fenfluramine (interaction may trigger serotonin syndrome)
		  Indirect sympathomimetics (interaction can result in hypertensive crisis)
		  Selective serotonin reuptake inhibitors (interaction may trigger serotonin syndrome)
		
		Interaction may result in dangerously high blood pressure:
		  Buspirone
		  L-dopa
		  Stimulants
		
		Patients also need to know that combining MAOIs and cocaine is extremely dangerous

and MAOIs[8–10]. The interaction between these drugs can be deadly. As a result, doctors try to ensure that patients have stopped taking the SSRI or MAOI and have eliminated the drug completely from their bodies before switching from one to the other. For example, it generally takes five times the half-life of an SSRI before the drug is out of a person's system[11]. Therefore, a patient taking the SSRI fluoxetine (Prozac®) will need to wait at least 5 weeks before starting an MAOI[10]. The waiting period will vary for each SSRI. Moving from an MAOI to an SSRI usually requires a 2-week waiting period[10,12].

If moderate to severe symptoms resembling serotonin syndrome are experienced, the patient should stop taking all antidepressant medications and immediately contact a medical doctor or go to a hospital emergency room. If one or more symptoms occur but are mild and inconvenient or annoying rather than causing moderate to severe difficulties, the patient should contact and follow the prescribing doctor's advice. Treatment for serotonin syndrome includes stopping the medication and providing medical care for the patient and support for the family. Patients in extreme distress or a fragile physical condition may require admission to an intensive-care unit. Doctors can also employ benzodiazepines, cyproheptadine, chlorpromazine, methysergide, and propranolol for treating the syndrome. Bromocriptine, a drug used for treating neuroleptic malignant syndrome, can worsen serotonin syndrome symptoms[13].

All antidepressants carry some risk for starting or increasing mania. While tricyclic drugs appear to

> **All antidepressants carry some risk for starting or increasing mania**

have a higher probability for triggering mania and rapid cycling than do MAOIs, SSRIs, and bupropion, none of the available antidepressants can safely be used singly as monotherapy for treating bipolar depression[14–16]. As a result, treatment guidelines developed by research and expert panels strongly recommend against using any class of antidepressants as a singular, stand-alone treatment for bipolar depression[17]. For some patients, antidepressants almost immediately start a hypomanic episode, while others initially receive symptom relief but then transition into a mixed bipolar depression[18]. This presents a paramount question for patients and doctors. If symptoms of depression appear before any history of manic or hypomanic episodes, how can a physician determine that the person may have a bipolar disorder and avoid employing a standard antidepressant monotherapy?

Unfortunately, this question does not have a good answer. Doctors are forced to make decisions based on the family's psychiatric history, symptom patterns, and hints from the person's current and past behaviors.

Some indicators such as racing thoughts, anger, and hallucinations are relatively easy to identify. Other symptoms and historical information are often less obvious, and sometimes unknown by the patient. Hypomanic episodes during adolescence or even young adulthood, for example, may have been dismissed and accepted as youthful energy. The patient and family may be so focused on the current depression that even when hypomanic symptoms are briefly explained, they do not cognitively link them to behaviors and events in the person's past. Furthermore, because descriptive words are differentially processed, understanding of their meaning, ability to stimulate memory, and create connections

---

Are Selective Serotonin Reuptake Inhibitors (SSRIs) Dangerous for Adult Patients With a Bipolar Disorder?

Many patients with bipolar disorders can safely take SSRIs when combined with a mood-stabilizing medication and closely supervised by a psychiatrist.

Research indicates the following:
* SSRIs are not recommended as monotherapy for depression related to bipolar disorder.
* SSRIs are not recommended in combination with monoamine oxidase inhibitor (MAOI) medications (see wash-out period before introducing an SSRI after patient has been on an MAOI).
* Evidence is mixed, but suggests that SSRIs may increase suicidal behaviors in children and adolescents.

between the past and present are highly variable from person to person.

It is difficult for people to identify or recall the difference between elevated mood and exaggerated self-esteem and spontaneity, especially in youths. Therefore, the significance of mental health professionals conducting a robust, slow assessment of past and present hypomanic symptoms cannot be overemphasized. It is helpful not only to provide numerous examples of hypomanic behavior, but also to assist patients in cognitively processing, discussing, and labeling how each behavioral example is like or different from their personal experiences. Family histories can also be difficult for patients to remember accurately and communicate clearly. In addition to social stigma causing people to hide psychiatric problems even within families since World War II, we live in an ever-increasingly mobile society. A growing number of people have had only distant relationships with second-generation family members and little or no knowledge of their family's third generation. As a result, families need help in learning how to discuss mental illness with distant relatives and identifying behavioral 'hints' of hidden and untreated disorders. Because psychiatric histories and symptoms are seldom straightforward, the diagnostic discovery process has to be a cooperative effort between the patient, treatment team, and family. Until a definitive biological marker for bipolar disorders is discovered, patients must rely on the medication knowledge and judgment of their doctors. This process will never be foolproof, but becomes more accurate when a complete and open communication flow exists between patients, families, and physicians.

MEDICATION TREATMENT FOR BIPOLAR MAJOR DEPRESSIVE EPISODES

At some point, every person with bipolar I disorder will have a major depression. The National Institute of Mental Health's prospective natural history study of bipolar disorders discovered that depression is more pervasive and common than mania. The 12.8-year study found that bipolar symptoms were present for 47% of the total patients' days, and depression accounted for two-thirds of these symptomatic days[19,20]. The overwhelming difficulty caused by depression for patients with bipolar disorder was also documented by Post and colleagues. Following patients from the Stanley Foundation network, these researchers found that patients had three times more problems with depression than with mania[21]. Together, these and other reports document that, compared with mania, bipolar depressive symptoms occur more often, last longer, and for many patients cause more disruptions in their family, work, school, community, and social functioning[20]. Therefore, the importance of encour-

---

Indicators of Possible Bipolar Disorder Before a Manic Episode Has Occurred

The following indicators may signal that a patient has a bipolar depression rather than a unipolar depression[2,3]:

- The patient's family has a history of bipolar disorder.
- The patient comes from three consecutive generations with mood disorders.
- Hypersomnia (excessive sleepiness) and psychomotor retardation more often appear in patients with bipolar depression than in those with unipolar depression.
- Onset often occurs at a younger age than in unipolar depression.
- Depressive episodes may occur closer together than in unipolar depression, causing more depressive episodes than expected in a defined period of time: depression recurs more often than expected.
- The patient may report depressive episodes that last less than 2 weeks in duration.
- Unlike unipolar depression, the patient fails to recover completely after depressive episodes.
- The depressed patient reports racing thoughts.
- Anger is pronounced and intense.
- Even though depressed, the patient seeks thrills and excitement.
- Sexual interest increases during a depressive episode.
- The depressed patient demonstrates mood-incongruent psychotic symptoms or hallucinations.

Improving the Initial Medication Assessment

Identifying bipolar depression that precedes manic symptoms is extremely difficult, requiring active participation from the patient, family, and physician. The following are suggestions to promote improved communications and facilitate medication decisions.

It is helpful if patients experiencing the onset of depression:

- Allow family or significant others to participate in the assessment and freely provide information and interpretations of the person's current and historical behaviors;
- Attempt, prior to the assessment, to discover if any first-, second-, or third-generation family members had mental illness;
- Identify whether, for the past three generations, any family members were not said to be mentally ill as such but were constantly noted for being 'odd', different, shy, 'hyper', or behaviorally strange (the lack of mental health resources and the stigma of mental disorders have prevented many from receiving needed assistance);
- Understand that diagnosing and assessing requires a doctor or therapist to evaluate how a person's behaviors, emotions, and social functioning have or have not changed within multiple community, family, and work settings;
- Know that the first episodes of bipolar depression can occur even though there are no current or historical indicators of vulnerability for bipolar disorders;
- Understand that early indicators of bipolar vulnerabilities do not necessarily mean that the depression will become a bipolar disorder;
- Even though feeling tired and perhaps agitated from depression, attempt to concentrate, participate in the assessment, and recall examples of past and current behaviors.

It is helpful if the diagnosing physician or therapist:

- Talks with and listens closely to the patient's concerns, self-descriptors, what is and is not emphasized, and hints about issues that are difficult for the individual to talk about;
- Attempts to help the patient discover and verbalize forgotten, overlooked life experiences that may seem unimportant to the person;
- Discusses and gains the family's or significant others' perspectives of the patient's strengths, symptoms, illness history, copying style, support systems, life situation and problems willingness and ability to follow treatment recommendations correctly and use of substances and over-the-counter medications;
- Discovers what the family knows about depression, mania, and bipolar disorders, what they are experiencing in the way of hardships, fears, and other concerns, what they have as concrete support systems, and what they need immediately in order to care for themselves and the patient;
- Develops a process that weaves education and assessment questions into an understandable gestalt and mutual discussion;
- Overcomes the patient's concentration difficulties by providing information and asking questions in shorter but connected cognitive chains;
- Slows the assessment process and helps the patient to understand better and recall possible hypomanic behaviors;
- Looks for cross-family agreement of past and current hypomanic behaviors;
- Attempts to inform and inquires about hypomanic symptoms in a manner that does not predispose responses from the patient ofrfamily;
- Receives consultation when a patient has an unusual history or complicated symptoms, or the mental health professional has only limited experience in diagnosing bipolar depression.

aging and supporting patients at their first sign of depression to seek professional medical help immediately cannot be overstated.

When experiencing the first onset of depression, many patients and families simply fail to recognize the symptoms as the start of a real illness, hope their situation will spontaneously improve, or attempt to resolve the problem by the use of herbal medications, increased alcohol intake, exercise, avoidance and attitude changes, or other home remedies. Patients who have previously experienced depression may hesitate to seek medical help, fearing hospitalization, or having concerns that child-protection services will remove their children or insist on close supervision and accountability. Fears of medication side-effects, social stigma, and family disapproval of drug therapy can also prevent patients from quickly returning to their psychiatrist. There is growing evidence that, when left untreated, depressive episodes increase in duration and the length of time between episodes decreases[6]. Therefore, families, friends, community workers, and employers need to join in a coordinated effort to encourage and persuade individuals to overcome their resistance and fears and quickly accept medical help.

While antidepressant monotherapy presents an unacceptable danger, the physician is not without a number of alternatives. Today, thanks to research, patients can be optimistic that a growing number of new medications and drug combinations will decrease their depressive episodes and lengthen the time between episodes (Table 6.3). As emphasized earlier, while science has yet to find a medical cure for bipolar disorders, advances are being made that offer hope for better control and management of the illness. Both research and expert review panels strongly recommend that the first line of treatment for bipolar depression be a mood stabilizer[22,23]. Treatment guidelines published by the World Federation of Societies of Biological Psychiatry recommend, for example, combining a mood stabilizer such as lithium or lamotrigine with an SSRI or bupropion antidepressant[24]. North American and European treatment guidelines differ principally in recommendations around the use of antidepressants for bipolar depression. United States researchers tend to have less confidence in quickly prescribing treatments that combine mood stabilizers and antidepressant medications, compared with European doctors[26].

Generally, the mood-stabilizing drugs most often used alone, or in combination with other medications, for controlling depressive and manic symptoms are lithium carbonate (brand names include Eskality®, Lithonate®, and Cibalith-S®), lamotrigine (brand name Lamictal®), divalproex sodium (also known as semisodium valproate, brand name Depakote®), sodium valproate (brand name Depakene®), valproic acid, and carbamazepine (brand names Tegretol®, Carbartol®, and Atretol®) (Table 6.4). All of the antimanic medications with the exception of lithium were originally developed

Table 6.3 Doses of medications used for acute-phase treatment* of bipolar depression. Reproduced from reference 25

Type/class	Medication	Usual target dose (mg/day)	Usual maximum recommended dose (mg/day)	Recommended administration schedule
Anticonvulsant	Lamotrigine	200[†]	600	q.d.
	Lithium			
Selective serotonin reuptake inhibitors	citalopram	20–40	60	q.d.
	fluoxetine	20	80	q.d.
	fluvoxamine	150–250	250	q.d.
	paroxetine	20	60	q.d.
	sertraline	50	200	q.d.
Others	bupropion	300	400	b.i.d.
	nefazodone	300–600	600	q.d.
	venlafaxine	150	375	b.i.d. or t.i.d.
	venlafaxine XR	75	225	q.d.

* Doses for maintenance treatment may be lower. [†]See manufacturer's recommendations for instructions for starting this medication; rapid and improper titration places patient at risk of serious side-effects. q.d., every day; b.i.d., twice a day; t.i.d., three times a day

and continue to be used as anticonvulsant medications.

Lithium is an element found in mineral springs, seawater, and certain rocks and ores. The naturally occurring lithium compounds are not directly suitable as drugs, and therefore for therapeutic use lithium is most often combined with carbonate ion in the form of lithium carbonate. Lithium was the first medication used effectively as a mood stabilizer for bipolar disorders. In the 1940s, John F.J. Cade, an Australian medical doctor and psychiatrist, believed that manic depression (today referred to as bipolar illness) was primarily a biological disorder. He discovered the therapeutic properties of lithium while researching whether the urine of manic–depressive patients contained unusual toxic compounds. His research called for injecting guinea-pigs with uric acid, a product of nucelic acid breakdown found in urine. Uric acid does not easily dissolve in water. To overcome this difficulty, Cade combined the uric acid with a lithium ion and water to form lithium urate. The uric acid injected into the animals as lithium urate seemed to be less harmful. As a result, Cade hypothesized that lithium served as a protective element against the uric acid. To test his idea, lithium carbonate was injected into the guinea-pigs. To Cade's surprise, within about 2 h the animals became unusually calm, lethargic, and unresponsive to their environment. This finding inspired Cade to use lithium for treating a number of patients suffering with severe mania. The results were startlingly dramatic. Patients who had been unable to function outside a hospital ward were experiencing normal moods and returning to society.

Table 6.4 Generic and brand names of mood-stabilizing medications

Generic name	Brand name
Lithium carbonate	Eskality®
	Lithonate®
	Cibalith-S®
Lamotrigine	Lamictal®
Divalproex sodium	Depakote®
Sodium valproate	Depakene®
Carbamazepine	Tegretol®
	Carbatol®
	Atretol®

Sadly, although documented in professional journals and talks, these findings were not quickly embraced by the mental-health professions. Some of the factors that delayed the development and adoption of lithium were scientific while others were political and economic. Immediately after World War II in Great Britain and the United States, psychiatry and mental health professionals as a whole embraced psychoanalytical concepts, and in Germany and Eastern Europe psychiatric practice and research was at a standstill. Finally in the late 1950s, Danish researchers led by Mogens Schou performed the necessary research to discover recommended dosages and requirements for using lithium safely. This moved the drug into general professional awareness during the 1960s and into use throughout the United States in the early 1970s[2,27,28].

In addition to establishing lithium as an effective treatment drug, Schou is also credited with empirically demonstrating that for some patients lithium has the ability to prevent future depressive and manic episodes[30].

Interestingly, lithium, the most traditional and widely used drug for controlling mania, is also effective in many patients for decreasing depressive symptoms. Studies indicate that lithium is effective for 30–79% of patients experiencing bipolar depression[22,23,31]. In a study using only lithium to treat bipolar depression, Goodwin and colleagues found that half of the sample experienced reduced symptoms and approximately one-third reported complete remission from depression (Figure 6.4)[32,33].

A problem with these early studies is that the samples included patients who had histories of either hypomania or major manic episodes. Nonetheless, a 1993 literature review found that eight out of nine placebo-controlled trials of lithium with patients who had bipolar I or bipolar II between 1960 and 1979 demonstrated that lithium was far superior to placebo for treating bipolar depression[23]. The review also included five studies that identified specifically whether patients had a complete or partial remission of depressive symptoms. Across these studies, lithium, as a single or monotherapy, successfully ended all major depression symptoms for 36% of patients[23]. Because of these and other research findings, the American Psychiatric Association's (APA) 2004 Practice Guidelines strongly endorse initially using lithium or the anticonvulsant lamotrigine for treating bipolar depression[17]. After reviewing perti-

A Short History of Lithium[2,7,29]

- The second-century Greek physician Seranus Ephisios recommended natural waters from alkaline springs for treating mania-like symptoms. Alkaline springs have been found to be rich in lithium.
- Roman physicians continued the Greek method of having patients with mental and physical problems drink and bathe in waters from selected pools.
- European countries throughout the centuries have used natural spas, many now known to be rich in lithium, for treating physical and mental disorders.
- In the 19th century gout and kidney stones were unsuccessfully treated with lithium.
- In the mid- to late 1940s, John F. J. Cade, MD started experimenting with lithium.
- In 1949 Dr Cade's research demonstrated that lithium successfully treated mania.
- In the late 1940s lithium was tragically used as a salt substitute for patients with heart disease, high blood pressure, and other medical problems, resulting in numerous lithium poisonings and several deaths.
- Lithium became extremely unpopular and questioned after the salt substitute tragedy, which may have played a role in delaying its use as a drug for treating bipolar disorders.
- Mid-1940s British and American psychiatric training programs and clinics embraced psychoanalytical theory and questioned the value of using medications for treating mental illness.
- During the mid-1940s the end of World War II left mental health research in Germany and much of Eastern Europe in disarray.
- German experimentation on Jews and prisoners caused many to reject research that 'altered' brain functioning and helped to reinforce psychoanalytical explanations for mental disorders.
- 1950s Danish researchers led by Mogens Schou systematically researched the properties, dose requirements, and safe management of lithium for treating bipolar disorders.
- In the 1960s lithium received general acceptance within the psychiatric community.
- In 1967 Mogens Schou and associates empirically demonstrated that lithium not only treats bipolar symptoms but for some patients prevents future depressive and manic episodes.
- By the 1970s lithium became the first line of treatment for bipolar disorders throughout the United States.
- From the late 1960s to the present, lithium was found to be effective for treating bipolar depression and caused fewer patients to switch into a manic episode compared with antidepressants.
- In the early 2000s lamotrigine was found to be more effective for treating bipolar depression than lithium.
- In the early 2000s lithium was found to be more effective for treating manic episodes than lamotrigine.

nent research studies, the APA Guidelines expressed substantial clinical confidence in lithium for treating bipolar depression and moderate confidence in the use of lamotrigine. As research documents lamotrigine's effectiveness and safety, future panels may give the drug a stronger recommendation.

Lamotrigine, developed by GlaxoSmithKline and marketed under the brand name Lamictal®, is the first medication since lithium to be approved by the United States Food and Drug Administration (FDA) for long-term maintenance treatment of patients with bipolar I disorder. The medication has shown effectiveness in delaying or preventing mania, hypomania, mixed episodes, and depression. Data from randomized studies indicates that lamotrigine is particularly robust in protecting patients from bipolar depression[34–36]. Moreover, an 18-month multicenter placebo-controlled study found that both lamotrigine and lithium delayed the onset of mood episodes, but lamotrigine was more effective in preventing depressive episodes[37]. Additionally, lamotrigine used as a monotherapy for depressive and manic episodes did not increase symptoms or accelerate mood cycling. The researchers found that

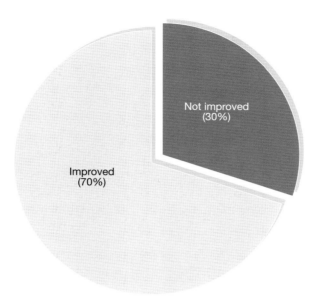

Figure 6.4 Results of lithium treatment for manic symptoms

approximately 4.6–5.4% of research patients treated for bipolar depression with only lamotrigine switched into either a hypomanic or a manic episode, compared with 5% of patients on placebo[35,37,38]. Additionally, there is evidence from a small study that lamotrigine is an effective monotherapy for bipolar II depressive and manic symptoms. The study compared patient functioning and symptoms for 6 months on lamotrigine and an SSRI, and for 6 months on just lamotrigine therapy. While on lamotrigine monotherapy, the patient group had significantly fewer depressive and manic episodes, episodes were shorter in duration, and psychosocial functioning as measured by the Global Assessment of Functioning (GAF) scale increased[39]. Even though these results are extremely promising, a definitive statement about lamotrigine's effectiveness as a monotherapy for bipolar II disorders cannot be given until further research is completed.

In addition to this drug's apparent effectiveness in treating bipolar I and II depression, there is also evidence that, compared with placebo, long-term use of lamotrigine does not cause patients to experience significant body weight gain. There is also preliminary evidence that lamotrigine causes fewer tremors and cognitive problems compared with lithium[40–42]. Lithium can cause subtle neurocognitive impairment in psychomotor speed, immediate and delayed verbal memory, and other executive functions[43]. It is less clear whether lithium used for maintenance interferes with attention and concentration. There is no evidence, however, that lithium taken as a long-term maintenance therapy causes ongoing cumulative neurocognitive damage[44]. While lamotrigine does not appear to decrease neurocognitive functioning, in rare cases it can cause a serious skin rash. A multicenter study reported that more patients on lamotrigine developed rashes than did individuals on

---

Lamotrigine Overview

- Lamotrigine is an anticonvulsant medication.
- It is FDA-approved (2003) as a long-term maintenance drug for treating chronic bipolar symptoms.
- It has been found to be effective for controlling and decreasing bipolar depression.
- The rate of medication-triggered mood switching is low and similar to placebo.
- Lamotrigine is more effective than lithium for controlling bipolar depression.
- It is effective for treating mania, but less so than lithium.

a placebo. However, the number of rashes in each group was similar and statistically insignificant[45].

The promise of decreased medication side-effects can tempt consumers to push for an immediate change in their drug therapy. Before advocating for a change to the medication regimen, patients should be asked the following questions:

(1) How stable have your bipolar symptoms been over the past 2–3 months?

(2) Are you currently in the midst of an episode?

(3) How many depressive and manic episodes have you had in the past 12–18 months?

(4) What has been your level of functioning at work or school and within the family and community over the past 12–18 months? Another way of thinking about this question is, over the past year, how do your social, communication, thinking, and work skills compare with before the onset of illness, or when you are at your best point of functioning?

(5) How stable is your current environment? Are you facing a personal, family, financial, or other type of crisis?

(6) How difficult or severe are the side-effects caused by your current medications?

(7) All medications have side-effects; therefore, how much do you really know and understand about lamotrigine's side-effects?

(8) Are you overweight more because of medication side-effects or because of your eating and exercise habits?

(9) What benefits will changing to lamotrigine provide other than possibly slowing your weight gain?

(10) Are you aware that lamotrigine is not a diet pill, that is, it does not cause people to gain weight, but it does not automatically reduce your current body weight?

(11) Why is your doctor either not advocating a change in your medications or not enthusiastic about switching to a different medication?

By answering such questions, consumers are reminded that medication treatment is a collaborative effort between the patient, the doctor, and, often, the family. Frequently, it is not wise to change

medications to lessen side-effects if you have remained stable and highly functional on your current drug therapy.

Furthermore, switching drugs during a period of personal crisis or difficulty can create additional stress and adjustment problems. If changes to medications are being considered, patients are encouraged to be certain that they can answer critical specific questions about why the change is wanted or advised by a doctor. Patients also need to be aware that certain illness profiles appear to respond better to lithium than to lamotrigine. At least one study has reported that people who respond better to lithium appear to be free of comorbid illnesses, and have more classical symptoms and fewer annual episodes. Those who do better on lamotrigine more often have rapid cycling and other atypical symptoms, an early age of illness onset, and an additional psychiatric disorder along with their bipolar illness[46].

While monotherapy with an anticonvulsant drug or with lithium is helpful, patients with more severe depressive episodes or a history of enduring difficult-to-treat bipolar depression may benefit from taking both a mood stabilizer and either an antidepressant or an antipsychotic medication. Combined therapy may also help some patients to continue their maintenance drug therapy. Bowden and Singh report that after 12–18 months of monotherapy with lithium, or divalproex, or lamotrigine, or olanzapine, only about 30% of patients reported having control of their illness, avoided new depression or manic episodes, or did not discontinue their medication because of uncomfortable side-effects. Combination drug therapy allows some patients to take lower medication dosages than required in monotherapy. Bowden and Singh's literature review found that an added drug is almost always given in a lower dosage than when prescribed as a monotherapy[3]. This may lessen side-effects and help patients to stay on their maintenance therapy regimen. Additionally, a single medication may address all of the problems and disruptions caused by bipolar disorders. For example, a patient may simultaneously have 4–6 major problems stemming from multiple brain areas. In such complex cases a single medication normally cannot control differing severe or even subtle symptoms[47].

Polydrug therapy is generally administered in one of two ways. In the 'add-on' method one medication is started and the second added after the person has adjusted to the initial drug. In treating bipolar depression it is important always to start with the mood stabilizer, determine the therapeutic benefits gained from the monotherapy, and then add the antidepressant. Starting with the antidepressant may trigger a switch to mania[3]. Also, it is important to determine the effectiveness of the mood stabilizer before adding additional medications. In some cases where time is an issue or the depression is extremely severe and worsening, doctors may want to prescribe an immediate 'co-therapy' and start the two different medications together. Virtually all combination drug studies have used the add-on approach, and little or no support exists in the psychiatric literature for using the co-therapy or concurrent method for treating bipolar disorders. Unfortunately, guidelines have not been established directing the amount of time needed before the second add-on medication is started[3]. As a result, doctors must rely on experience, clinical urgency, patient and family reports, and the known time required before a drug's benefits start before prescribing the second medication.

COMBINING MOOD STABILIZERS AND ANTIDEPRESSANTS

If lithium alone fails to control bipolar depression, an SSRI, MAOI, norepinephrine and dopamine reuptake inhibitor (NDRI), or other drug is often add to the treatment regimen. In combination with lithium or other mood stabilizers, the risk of antidepressants switching patients into a hypomanic or manic episode is markedly lowered (Figure 6.5). This is particularly true when the newer families of antidepressants such as SSRIs and NDRIs (bupropion) are used with a mood stabilizer[48]. Research indicates that modern antidepressants combined with mood stabilizers not only help to decrease depression but

also reduce the risk of medication-induced mania by approximately 50%[49–52]. There is also evidence that, in some cases, continuing to take an antidepressant medication after the remission of symptoms prevents or delays relapse without increasing the risk for inducing mania. A small study by researchers from the University of California at Los Angeles found that depressive episodes could be prevented or delayed by continuing combined antidepressant and mood-stabilizer medications after a depressive episode ended. This is routinely done in treating unipolar depression, but the risk of bipolar patients switching from depression to mania causes doctors to discontinue antidepressants more quickly.

The California researchers documented that within 1 year, 70% of all individuals who stopped using an antidepressant immediately after their symptoms lifted relapsed back into depression. If, however, the antidepressant and mood stabilizer combination was maintained for 6–12 months after symptom remission, relapse dropped to 53%, and if both medications were maintained for 12 or more months, at the end of 1 year only 24% of the group experienced a depressive episode. Furthermore, the study also found that reduced time on an antidepressant is associated with a greater risk for switching from depression to mania. Within 1 year, a manic episode was experienced by:

(1) 29% of patients who discontinued antidepressant treatment immediately after depressive symptoms ended;

(2) 22% who continued both an antidepressant and antimanic medication for 6–12 months;

(3) 5% of patients who remained on the combined drugs for 12 or more months[53].

Treating Mixed Episodes and Rapid Cycling

Mixed episodes and rapid cycling do not always respond to lithium as robustly as do classical bipolar depression and mania. Research and expert panels recommend that if a mixed episode or rapid cycling does not respond to lithium, or the person cannot take lithium during an acute episode, the following medications and treatments should be considered:
- Divalproex sodium;
- Lamotrigine;
- Carbamazepine;
- Antimanic drug combinations;
- Electroconvulsive therapy.

The findings provide a logical argument for extending the time that antidepressants are employed for treating bipolar depression. While this is an important study, it has a number of limitations. As an example, the research participants were not randomly selected, and knew exactly when the antidepressant was discontinued. A preponderance of psychopharmacology literature underscores that even though SSRIs and bupropion appear to be safer than tricyclic medications, the majority of research continues to place suspicion on long-term use of all antidepressants for treating bipolar depression[54]. Problems that are commonly associated with taking three different types of non-MAOI antidepressants are listed in Table 6.5.

Therefore, until a robust study documents the efficacy of long-term antidepressant treatment for bipolar disorders, mental health professionals and consumers should use the above findings with caution.

TREATING MANIC EPISODES

Manic episodes are dangerous for patients and disruptive for families. As the first symptoms of agitation, aggression, impulsivity, delusional thinking, or hallucinations appear, treatment must be assertively and systematically initiated. Identifying the start of a manic episode is often difficult. Few patients start or remain in a state of euphoria and grandiosity for an extended period of time. Studies indicate that during a manic episode, irritability, depression, and mood lability are experienced as much as or more than euphoria[1]. As with bipolar depression, medications are the first line of treat-

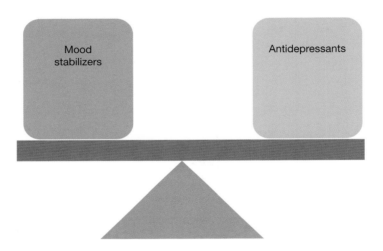

Figure 6.5 Balancing mood stabilizers and antidepressants can prevent mania for some patients

Table 6.5 Side-effects of non-MAOI antidepressants

	Fluoxetine (Prozac®) – on SSRI	Imipramine (Tofranil®) – on TCA	Bupropion (Wellbutrin®) – on NDRI
Agitation, insomnia	common	uncommon	common
Blurry vision, constipation, dry mouth	uncommon	common	uncommon
Gastrointestinal distress, diarrhea	common	uncommon	uncommon
Sedation, drowsiness	uncommon	common	uncommon
Weight gain	uncommon	common	uncommon

MAOI, monoamine oxidase inhibitor; SSRI, selective serotonin reuptake inhibitor; TCA, tricyclic antidepressant; NDRI, norepinephrine and dopamine reuptake inhibitor

ment for hypomania and mania. Psychoeducation helps patients and families to identify signs that an episode is starting, but neither education nor psychotherapy provides effective treatment for hypomania or mania.

The most common drugs recommended by researchers and expert panels for treating acute mania are lithium, divalproex sodium, and antipsychotic medications. Monotherapy for mania using lithium, divalproex sodium, olanzapine, carbamazepine, ziprasidone, aripiprazole, or chlorpromazine has proven more effective than placebo[55,56]. Table 6.6 give recommended doses of these medications and Table 6.7 lists side-effects of three of them. Nonetheless, monotherapy for severe acute mania seldom quickly achieves complete remission of symptoms. As a result, practice guidelines for treating severe acute mania commonly call for using either lithium or divalproex sodium along with an antipsychotic. Patients with hypomania or moderate mania may respond positively to a monotherapy regimen of lithium, divalproex sodium, or an antipsychotic[15,53].

Lithium is the original antimanic medication and continues in wide use throughout the world. The drug works better for patients with classic manic episodes. Research continues to find this drug effective in adults for both treating and preventing acute mania and bipolar depression. Additionally, lithium appears to help stabilize and limit inappropriate moods between episodes[1]. For treating acute mania, lithium is often more effective when plasma concentrations are at the higher therapeutic level

(1.0–1.4 mmol/l)[57]. Lithium, lamotrigine, and olanzapine have been approved by the FDA for long-term maintenance treatment of bipolar disorders. Some professionals hypothesize that combining lithium and lamotrigine may improve maintenance treatment for patients who do not have mixed episodes or rapid cycling[20]. The therapeutic logic is based on studies indicating that lithium is more effective in treating classical mania than is lamotrigine, and lamotrigine appears to be better for intervening with bipolar depression than is lithium[37,40]. The hypothesis' efficacy has not yet been completely tested.

Divalproex sodium is approved by the FDA for treating acute mania. The drug's efficacy as a therapy for acute mania has been demonstrated in numerous research studies. It has been found to be superior in treating acute mania compared with placebo, and appears to give results that are similar to those with lithium. Some patients, however, report that divalproex sodium starts to relieve symptoms faster than lithium. While divalproex sodium results are comparable with lithium, people who either cannot tolerate or are refractory to lithium may have a positive treatment response with divalproex sodium[58]. The anticonvulsant may be more helpful than lithium for patients who experience repeated rapid mood swings and have mixed episodes where depression is more prominent than mania[57]. Additional studies are needed before a patient profile can be developed for advising who will best respond to divalproex sodium treatment.

Table 6.6 Summary of recommended doses of medications used for acute phase treatment* of mania/hypomania. Reproduced from reference 25

Type/class	Medication	Usual target dose (level)	Usual maximum recommended dose (level)	Recommended administration schedule
	Lithium	(0.8–1.0 mmol/l)	(1.2 mmol/l)	b.i.d. or q.h.s.
Anticonvulsants	oxcarbazepine	600–2100 mg/day	2400 mg/day	b.i.d. or t.i.d.
	divalproex sodium	(80 μg/ml)	(125 mg/ml)	b.i.d. or q.h.s.
Atypical antipsychotics	clozapine	100–300 mg/day	900 mg/day	q.h.s.
	olanzapine	10–15 mg/day	20 mg/day	b.i.d. or q.h.s.
	risperidone	2 mg/day	6 mg/day	b.i.d. or q.h.s.
	quetiapine	200–600 mg/day	800 mg/day	b.i.d. or q.h.s.
	ziprasidone	40–160 mg/day	160 mg/day	b.i.d.

*Doses used for maintenance treatment may be lower. b.i.d., twice a day; q.h.s., each bed-time; t.i.d., three times a day

Table 6.7 Side-effects of medications for bipolar disorder

	Divalproex sodium (Depakote®)	Lithium	Carbamazepine (Tegretol®)
Common	drowsiness	diarrhea	dizziness
	nausea	nausea	drowsiness
		skin rashes	
		tremors	
		urinary changes	
		weight gain	
Uncommon	accidental injury	aggressiveness	abnormal bleeding
	dizziness	anxiety	blurred vision
	skin rashes	blurred vision	constipation
		heat or cold intolerance	dry mouth
		memory problems	gastric distress
		mood changes	high fever
			infection
			nausea
			pigmentation in eyes
			urinary changes

In at least one study there was no association between the effectiveness of the drug for reducing acute mania and in patients with mixed episodes or rapid cycling[58,59]. A multicenter study found that divalproex sodium, but not lithium, was associated with reducing acute manic symptoms for patients with a history of numerous previous episodes. It is not clear whether the results can be extended to maintenance treatment for mania[60]. Moreover, adding divalproex sodium to lithium when patients are not responding to lithium as a monotherapy may provide a more positive outcome[61]. There is little evidence that divalproex sodium provides effective monotherapy for maintenance of mania. However, future studies may continue to document the role of divalproex sodium in long-term maintenance treatment when combined with other medications. In addition, the medication appears to treat both manic and psychotic symptoms. No significant difference was found in the improvement of psychotic symptoms from studies comparing divalproex sodium with neuroleptic medications[62-64]. Similar results were achieved when patients were treated with either divalproex sodium or olanzapine, an atypical antipsychotic medication[64,65].

Olanzapine (Zyprexa®), manufactured by Eli Lilly, is a unique new-generation antipsychotic medication that is also effective for treating acute mania. The drug was approved in 2000 for treating acute mania and in 2004 for maintenance treatment of bipolar illness. This is the third drug approved by the FDA for treating acute mania and is associated with positive responses in patients with and without psychosis. In the United States, Symbyax®, a drug combining olanzapine and fluoxetine has received FDA approval for treating bipolar depression. A multicenter study of 833 patients found that the combination drug proved significantly superior to placebo and olanzapine monotherapy. Between weeks 4 and 8, patients taking the combination drug experienced greater improvement than those on olanzapine alone[66]. The project included patients with and without histories of psychoses. Approximately 19% of the participants experienced weight gain. This was a randomized double-blind study sponsored by the drug's manufacturer. In the future, it would be helpful for researchers to maintain patients on the combination treatment for an extended period of time. The 8-week study is impressive and provides hope for treating bipolar I depression. However, a longer maintenance period is needed to determine which patients have higher positive response rates, and whether the combination causes certain patients over time to destabilize into a manic episode. Because olanzapine is effective for treating both mania and psychosis, the drug gains importance when it is not clear whether a patient has bipolar disorder or schizophrenia.

Both the American Psychiatric Association[17] and the Texas Medication Algorithm Project (see below) state that olanzapine should be considered as a first-line option for treating acute bipolar mania. Specifically, treatment guidelines recommend a combination of a neuroleptic such as olanzapine and lithium or divalproex sodium for patients with severe acute mania. Patients with less severe mania may respond to olanzapine alone[17] The drug, however, consistently performs better than placebo. As an example, a study of 139 hospitalized patients with acute mania demonstrated that olanzapine is significantly better than placebo for improving acute manic symptoms, psychosis, and global functioning. In addition, a significantly higher proportion of the olanzapine-medicated in-patients were in the treatment-responding group. The study also documented that response was not dependent on symptom characteristics such as mixed episodes and rapid cycling[67,68]. This suggests, but does not prove, that olanzapine is effective across a wide spectrum of bipolar symptoms and subtypes.

In addition to treating acute mania, olanzapine can also be used as a maintenance treatment for bipolar illness. For some patients, the drug has been found to speed recovery. This was illustrated in a 47-week double-blind study comparing olanzapine with divalproex sodium. The group administered olanzapine had quicker and better overall remission of manic symptoms, but the rate of relapse did not significantly differ between the two drugs[63]. Nonetheless, olanzapine has been successfully used in the maintenance phase as a monotherapy and in combination with divalproex sodium and lithium. Physicians may especially want to consider using olanzapine for maintenance when a patient has a history of relapsing into psychosis, or cannot tolerate, or does not respond to lithium or other antimania medications. There is also some evidence that olanzapine is effective with children and adolescents who are in a manic episode. However, very few studies have been conducted with youth of any age, and all of the research has used only open trials of olanzapine or relied on retrospective records review[69].

ANTIPSYCHOTIC DRUGS

Standard or typical neuroleptic medications have long been used for treating acute mania, but are less than effective and to some extent dangerous for long-term bipolar maintenance therapy. For example, a 2-year maintenance study found that patients taking only lithium did as well as those on lithium and a standard antipsychotic drug[70]. Standard neuroleptic medications also have the added deficit of being associated with tardive dyskinesia. This is a drug-induced movement disorder that patients with bipolar disorders may be more susceptible to than other psychiatric patient groups[69,71]. Fortunately, a new generation of more effective and often safer atypical antipsychotic medications is now available. The APA Practice Guidelines state that the new generation of atypical antipsychotic medications is preferred for treating manic and mixed bipolar episodes over typical antipsychotic drugs. Research evidence, according to the APA Guidelines, supports the use of olanzapine or risperidone for treating bipolar disorders over the other atypical and all typical antidepressant drugs[17].

A critical review of research studies by Yatham found that the atypical antipsychotic medications olanzapine, risperidone, and quetiapine have efficacy as monotherapies for acute mania. Only minor differences in effectiveness were found among the three drugs when used as treatment for acute mania. Combined with a mood stabilizer, the three atypical antipsychotic drugs appear to gain in effectiveness and increase the number of people responding positively by about 20%. Furthermore, Yatham found no evidence across all of the reviewed studies that any of the atypical antidepressants triggered or increased the severity of depressive or manic symptoms[69].

Only one study has directly compared olanzapine with a first-generation typical antipsychotic drug. In-patients with acute mania were placed on either haloperidol ($n = 219$) or olanzapine ($n = 234$). The project started as an open-label study and then at the midpoint switched to a double-blind design. Halfway through the 12-week study there was no difference between the two groups' treatment responses. This changed dramatically by the study's final week. As the study ended, significantly more patients in the olanzapine group were in remission (68% vs. 41%). Furthermore, depression symptoms in general, and patients without a psychosis, responded significantly better to olanzapine than to the first-generation

---

Should Medications be Taken While Pregnant?

Managing bipolar disorders during pregnancy is a difficult task. All medications create some risk for the fetus. However, plunging into a severe depressive or manic episode is risky for both the mother and the fetus. As explained in Chapter 5, the risk for suicide and accidental harm increases as depression and mania symptoms worsen. The decision to take or discontinue medications during pregnancy is best determined through conversations between the mother, her family, and the treating psychiatrist. Principally, one needs to know the level and type of risk created by taking psychotropic drugs while pregnant. The following are a few facts and issues that a patient should be aware of and discuss with her doctor[1,73]:

- Certain medications can cause a developing fetus to be born with a malformed body or damaged internal organs.
- Delivery problems related to the medications may occur.
- Medications can cause hidden problems that later result in or influence behavior, learning, or psychiatric problems for the child.
- Mothers are normally advised to stop lithium during the first 3 months of pregnancy.
- During pregnancy many doctors advise against treating mild mania, but support treating more severe episodes.
- Electroconvulsive therapy can be used for treating mania without harming the fetus.

---

typical antipsychotic medication. The haloperidol group experienced significantly more extrapyramidal side-effects, and patients on olanzapine gained significantly more weight[72]. This provides important documentation that the new atypical antipsychotic medications in general, and olanzapine specifically, better protect patients from extrapyramidal side-effects and provide a more robust treatment for manic and depressive symptoms.

Olanzapine's chemical structure is related to that of clozapine, which was the first of the new-generation antipsychotic medications. In treating bipolar symptoms, olanzapine is more potent and has clinical features differing from those of both risperidone and clozapine. For most people, the drug given at moderate and even high dosages does not cause extrapyramidal symptoms. Additionally, while olanzapine is mildly sedative, it is not associated with the extreme sedation problems reported for clozapine. Early studies also indicate that olanzapine has an unusually low incidence rate for triggering tardive dyskinesia. This is extremely important and reassuring for patients who must take an antipsychotic medication for long extended periods of time. Surveys indicate that in an attempt to control mania 77–89% of patients with bipolar disorders take an antipsychotic medication[69]. Unfortunately, olanzapine's antihistaminic and serotonin 2C antagonist properties may cause patients to gain weight[6]. More

important, however, the FDA has requested all manufacturers of atypical antipsychotics to add warnings on their labels indicating that the medication is associated with an increased risk of hyperglycemia and diabetes. Additionally, using atypical antipsychotics in the elderly may increase the risk for strokes and death. Patients who have diabetes and take olanzapine need to receive increased routine monitoring from their doctor.

SUBSTANCE ABUSE AND BIPOLAR DISORDERS

Among psychiatric patients, individuals with bipolar I illness have one of the higher addiction rates. Epidemiological studies in the United States document that 46% of individuals with a bipolar disorder compared with 13% of the general population either abuse or are addicted to alcohol. Many of these individuals are also addicted to or abusing street drugs. Approximately 41% of people with bipolar disorders compared with 6% of the general public are thought to abuse street drugs[74,75]. The drug of choice is most often alcohol, but patients are also vulnerable to all addictive street drugs when in either a depressive or a manic episode[75]. Mania removes the person's inhibitions and insight into the danger of substance abuse, while depression stirs a search for ways to deaden psychological pain and overwhelming feelings of emptiness. There is a belief that using alcohol during bipolar episodes decreases the effectiveness of lithium. However, this remains an open question, because the combination of bipolar symptoms and substance abuse generally increases medication non-compliance and decreases one's ability to recall when and how the mood stabilizer was taken[1]. Obviously, adding alcohol or street drugs on top of depressive or manic symptoms has a high probability of increasing illness severity and multiplying a person's problems. Additionally, alcohol and street drugs can have effects that mimic bipolar symptoms. Alcohol may induce depressive behaviors and agitation while stimulants trigger symptoms that mirror mania. In addition to complicating diagnostic assessments, substance abuse may also increase the person's vulnerability for developing a more severe mental illness. Theoretically, alcohol and street drugs disrupt or create a harmful variation within the brain's chemistry, which has already been altered by the depressive or manic episodes. That is, substance abuse is thought to stress an already injured brain and increase the probability that the person will experience more severe or additional symptoms[76].

There is some evidence that lithium may actually help decrease alcohol use among people with a bipolar disorder. Unfortunately, the research in this area is very mixed and inconclusive[77-79]. Atypical antipsychotic drugs such as olanzapine and clozapine seem to help in decreasing alcohol abuse in patients with schizophrenia. The necessary research for determining the effectiveness of these medications in bipolar patients who abuse drugs has not been completed. There is also little evidence that anticonvulsants significantly curb substance abuse by patients with bipolar disorders[76]. Several steps are needed in treating patients with dual bipolar and substance abuse disorders. Generally, it is accepted that mood-stabilizing drugs have positive effects on bipolar symptoms even when the patient is abusing a substance. Therefore, it is important for families and clinicians to encourage substance-abusing patients to remain on their prescribed medications and, when possible, to supervise and ensure that the treatment medications are properly taken. However, medications need to be immediately stopped if a medical provider or pharmacist advises the patient that the illegal drug interacts dangerously with the prescribed medications. In addition to continuing medications, the patient will benefit from:

(1) Periodic substance-abuse education;

(2) Simultaneous and ongoing treatment for substance abuse and bipolar symptoms;

(3) Attending specialized self-help groups, that is, groups designed for people with bipolar disorders and cognizant that the treatment and support needed for such people who also abuse substances differ from what is required;

(4) Families trained to understand both bipolar disorders and substance abuse;

(5) Families trained to identify when a patient is vulnerable for abusing substances and to know how to get professional help as the person's risk factors increase;

(6) Added appointments with case managers or therapists as risk factors increase;

(7) Having a companion or family member present around the clock as risk factors increase;

(8) The ability to check into a partial hospital, day hospital, or in-patient unit as risk factors increase.

MEDICATIONS FOR CHILDREN AND YOUNG ADOLESCENTS WITH BIPOLAR DISORDERS

There is little doubt that a child or adolescent with a bipolar disorder needs medication treatment. Yet, few controlled studies have been performed to document the efficacy of drug treatment for children with bipolar disorders. Moreover, childhood bipolar disorder symptoms overlap with behaviors found in attention deficit, hyperactivity, and conduct disorders. These disorders are often treated with a stimulant medication. Rapid cycling can be triggered when a child with a bipolar disorder is misdiagnosed and placed on a stimulant or antidepressant[6]. Once correctly diagnosed, treatment for children and adolescents often starts with a regimen of either lithium or divalproex sodium. These two drugs appear to have been researched in youths more than the other leading medications. As in adults, divalproex sodium is often initiated in children who have rapid cycling or mixed episodes. Additional studies are needed, but atypical antipsychotic medications show promise for stabilizing moods in children and adolescents. Because of the lack of research, experts can make no recommendations for the use of anti-convulsant drugs with youths of any age[80].

There is evidence, however, that medications work in young patients. The only double-blind lithium study conducted with adolescents who had bipolar disorder and substance abuse showed significant improvement in their global functioning on lithium compared with placebo[81]. In an 18-month prospective study, relapse was experienced in 37% of adolescent participants who remained on lithium compared with 92% of teens who stopped their lithium[82]. A combination study using lithium and divalproex sodium with 102 children between the ages of 5 and 17 years demonstrated that the medication regimen significantly improved symptoms compared with the participants' baseline functioning[83]. In addition, a few small studies indicating effectiveness have been reported for the use of olanzapine, risperidone, quetiapine, and lamotrigine in

youths[80]. All of the studies, including those done with lithium, need to be replicated and better designed scientifically. The limited research helps to underscore that medications can relieve childhood bipolar symptoms, and that currently the initial treatment of choice is either a mood stabilizer or an antipsychotic medication. Children with more severe disorders may require a combination treatment. In these cases, lithium plus divalproex sodium, lithium plus olanzapine, or lithium plus carbamazepine are often prescribed[80]. Clinical experience shows that some children will need rather high medication doses during acute episodes. Therefore, it is imperative for parents and patients to understand that blood levels must be consistently checked and side-effects monitored[84]. Experts recommend that youths remain on a mood-stabilizing medication for a minimum of 2 years after their manic and depressive symptoms are in remission[80].

Table 6.8 Summary of levels of evidence for treating childhood mania

	Bipolar I disorder, manic or mixed without psychosis	Bipolar I disorder, manic or mixed with psychosis	Bipolar depressive episode
Lithium	A & B	A & B	B & C
Divalproex	B & C	B & C	C
Carbamazepine	B	B	ND
Oxcarbazepine	D	D	ND
Topiramate	C	C	ND
Clozapine	C	C	ND
Risperidone	B & C	B & C	ND
Olanzapine	B & C	B & C	B
Quetiapine	B & C	B & C	B
Ziprasidone	B & C	B & C	ND
Aripiprazole	B & C	B	ND
Selective serotonin reuptake inhibitors	NA	NA	C*
Bupropion	NA	NA	D
Lamotrigine	C	C	B & D

Level A data consist of child/adolescent placebo-controlled, randomized clinical trials. Level B data consist of adult randomized clinical trail. Level C data consist of open child/adolescent trials and retrospective analysis. Level D data consist of child/adolescent case reports or the panel consensus as to recommend current clinical practices. ND = no data. NA= not applicable. Reproduced with permission from reference 85. * May be mood destabilizing.

The above table summarizes the available research evidence for medication treatment with children and adolescents who have bipolar I disorder. Furthermore, the consensus panel agreed that when treating acute mania in youths level A drugs are given primacy over level B, level B has precedence over Level C, and Level C is preferred over Level D

BIPOLAR TREATMENT ALGORITHMS

An *algorithm* is a set of rules, guidelines, and defined steps that allow one to make decisions based on a logical flow of information. It is a tool for systematic problem-solving and decision-making. Torrey and Knable question whether an algorithm can be created for directing the treatment of bipolar disorders. These influential researchers argue correctly that inflexible one-dimensional algorithms cannot address a patient's individual needs. They emphasize that treatment for bipolar disorders must be a collaboration between the patient, doctor, and family[73].

Families, consumers, and mental health professionals have fought hard and long to reject or turn away from these principles. Nonetheless, there are also sound reasons for employing treatment algorithms, and methods of using best-practice guidelines that enhance the collaborative model. Among other things, a treatment algorithm can help to ensure that personal biases do not skew the assessment process, and that pertinent diagnostic and treatment decision steps are consistently and systematically considered. Furthermore, a well-designed algorithm allows input from all participants. It is a structure that can both detect the need for and accommodate exceptions. Numerous decision trees and algorithms have been designed over the years. One example currently being used by some clinicians and policy-makers was developed by the State of Texas. In order to support the understanding and use of the algorithm's logic, user requirements, and potential value, the Texas Medication Algorithm Project (TMAP) has placed their consumer information and physician's manual on the following World Wide Web site: http://www.mhmr.state.tx.us/centraloffice/medicald irector/TMAPtoc.html. The TMAP decision trees for helping doctors and patients make medication decisions for treating mania and depression are reproduced in Algorithms 1–4.

There are currently several studies and algorithms being developed to systematize and increase the use of evidence based practice for treating children with bipolar disorders. Hawaii has computerized the research studies for every major child disorder. This is an ongoing state-sponsored project that allows clinicians to have immediate access to research findings for guiding their intervention decisions. Minnesota is in the process of evaluating whether requiring the use a modified Hawaiian database for directing clinician decisions will significantly improve child treatment outcomes. Specific information about the Hawaiian model can be found on the web at http://www.state.hi.us/health/mental-health/ camhd/practice/ebs-index.html. Recently the *Journal of American Academy of Child and Adolescent Psychiatry* published algorithms for treating children with mania (Algorithms 1 and 2)[85]. The treatment guidelines were developed by having an expert panel review relevant research literature and reach a consensus around major treatment recommendations. This required evaluating and ranking the scientific evidence supporting most or all known medications available for treating childhood mania (Table 6.8). The panel also reminded clinicians that a number of medical conditions and medications can mimic or increase mood cycling in children and adolescents (Table 6.9)[85]. Obviously, successful use of algorithms and protocols is dependent on an accurate diagnosis and a comprehensive understanding of the patient's unique characteristics, culture, age, family, developmental history, and current social-economic situation.

Table 6.9 Medical conditions that may mimic mania or increase mood cycling in children and adolescents

Mimic mania

Temporal lobe epilepsy

Hyperthyroidism

Closed or open head injury

Multiple sclerosis

Systemic lupus erythematosus

Alcohol-related neurodevelopmental disorder

Wilson's disease

Increase mood cycling

Tricyclic antidepressants

Selective serotonin reuptake inhibitors

Serotonin and norepinephrine reuptake inhibitors

Aminophylline

Corticosteroids

Sympathomimetic amines (e.g. pseudoephedrine)

Antibiotics (e.g. clarithromycin, erythromycin, amoxicillin)

(Abouesh et al., 2002)

Reproduced with permission from reference 85.

Medical disorders and medications can mimic, increase, or trigger manic behaviors. Therefore, a comprehensive medical and medication histories are required as part of the child's diagnostic assessment

> Evidence based practice increasingly requires mental health professionals to incorporate algorithms, computerized protocols, and manualized interventions into their treatment of major mental disorders

Algorithm I Interpreting the Child Bipolar I Disorder Algorithm I. (Bipolar I disorder, manic or mixed, without psychosis)*

Stage 1   Monotherapy
High agreement was found among the expert panel for stage 1 interventions
First line of treatment is a monotherapy using traditional mood stabilizers or atypical antipsychotic medications
The lack of research evidence prevented making a definitive recommendation for which mood stabilizer or atypical antipsychotic drug should initially be prescribed to a youth with bipolar I illness
A majority of the panel however, recommended starting medication treatment for non-psychotic mania with lithium or divalproex
Selection of the initial stage 1 medication is dependent on the psychiatrist's experience in using the drugs, observed side-effects, and the child's overall reactions to the agent
The lack of research evidence prevented the inclusion of ziprasidone, aripiprazole, and oxcarbazepine in stage 1 monotherapy recommendations. Future findings may change this decision

Stage 1A   Monotherapy plus augmentation
The panel recommended prescribing an augmentation drug for children who partially improve from the monotherapy
When lithium is initially used as the monotherapy, doctors may consider adding divalproex, carbamazepine, olanzapine, quetiapine, or risperidone
If divalproex is used as a monotherapy the augmentation drug can be lithium, olanzapine, quetiapine, or risperidone
There was some support from the panel for combining lithium and divalproex before non-psychotic mania was treated with a combination that included an atypical antipsychotic medication
When a child has a partial response to a monotherapy with an atypical antipsychotic agent consider augmentation treatment with lithium, divalproex, or carbamazepine

Stage 2   Alternate monotherapy
If the initial monotherapy fails, or the drug cannot be tolerated, switch the monotherapy to one of the stage 1 medications that has not been previously prescribed
When there is no response to the augmentation drug initiate monotherapy with a medication that was not given in stage 1

Stage 2A   Alternate monotherapy plus augmentation
As in stage 1A, if the child has a partial response to the medication used in stage 2, consider augmentation treatment with a drug that was not prescribed in stage 1

Stages 3A   No definitive opinion was reached by panel members for treating children who fail to respond after being tried
and 3B   on two different monotherapy medications.
Part of the panel recommended selecting a third monotherapy medication that was not used in stages 1 or 2 (see stage 3A of algorithm)
Other panel members believed that a child who had not responded to previous monotherapy agents would not be helped by a third alternative monotherapy drug. These experts recommended using one of the combination drug treatment's listed in stage 3B of the algorithm

Stages 4A   Combination of two mood stabilizers or combination of three mood stabilizers
and 4B   Children who fail to respond or only partially respond to the monotherapy in stage 3A are candidates for treatment with two mood stabilizers
Recommended combinations are provided in stage 4A of the algorithm
If a child does not respond, or only has a partial response to augmentation with a monotherapy drug (stage 2A), or has no more than a partial response to treatment with two mood stabilizers (stage 3B), the combination drug treatments listed in stage 4B may be helpful

Stage 5   Alternate monotherapy
For stage 5 the panel recommended alternate monotherapy using oxcarbazepine, Ziprasidone, or Aripiprazole. It is important to note that as shown in Table 6.2 these drugs have only been studied using case reports or reviews by expert panels. Their efficacy with children and adolescents has not been researched using placebo-controlled, randomized clinical trials.

Algorithm for treating childhood manic or mixed episodes without psychosis

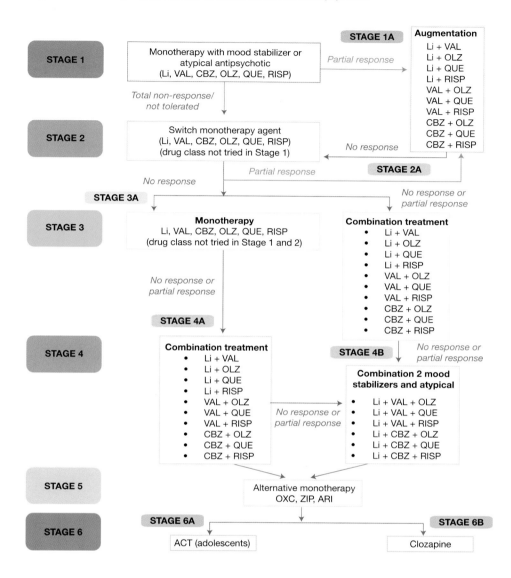

Algorithm 1

Gabapentin was not recommended for use with children and adolescents by the panel because the drug has failed to show efficacy in treating adults with mania

Lamotrigine was not recommended for treating acute manic episodes in youths. The panel could find no research that used lamotrigine to treat manic episodes in children and adolescents. As stated in other sections of this book lamotrigine has been found effective for maintenance treatment of adults with bipolar disorder I

Stage 6   Electroconvulsive therapy (ECT) or clozapine

Clozapine is recommended for children and adolescents who fail to respond to any of the treatments outlined in stages 1 to 5, or for youths who could not tolerate any of the above monotherapy agents or combination treatments

The panel recommended ECT only for adolescents. Children were not seen as candidates for ECT.

The use of ECT with adolescents has only been studied using case reports. ECT is reported to effectively treat acute mania in medication resistant adolescents. However, research using a more robust design has not been conducted

Because of insufficient data the panel could not determine if clozapine or ECT was more effective with medication resistant adolescents

*Summarized from reference 85

Algorithm 2 Interpreting the Child Bipolar I Disorder Algorithm II. (Bipolar I disorder, manic or mixed, with psychosis)*

Stage 1   Mood stabilizer plus atypical antipsychotic

The panel recommended that children who are diagnosed with bipolar disorder I, and have manic or mixed episodes and psychosis should initially be treated with a traditional mood stabilizer combined with an atypical antipsychotic medication

Open trial clinical research has shown lithium plus an atypical antipsychotic drug to be effective for treating acute mania and psychosis in adolescents

Based on clinical experience the panel recommended divalproex plus an atypical antipsychotic or a combination of carbamazepine and an atypical antipsychotic as optional interventions

Stage 1A   Augmentation

When children do not respond to stage 1 recommendations a combination of three medications (lithium + Divalproex + an atypical antipsychotic or lithium + Carbamazepine + an atypical antipsychotic medication) can be prescribed

This recommendation is based completely on case studies and reports by expert clinicians

Stage 2

When the child either fails to respond or cannot tolerate the regiment used in stage 1 the panel recommends prescribing a different untried stage 1 combination

Stage 2A

An augmentation drug is recommended when a mood stabilizer plus an atypical antipsychotic combination provides a partial response

This recommendation is based completely on case studies and reports by expert clinicians

Lithium, plus divalproex plus an atypical antipsychotic is an example of augmentation treatment

Stage 3   Mood stabilizer plus alternate

An alternate atypical antipsychotic may be added when the child fails to respond to a traditional mood stabilizer plus an atypical antipsychotic

As an example, the panel suggests that if lithium and risperidone are used in stage 2 with little or no success, the doctor may want to switch to lithium plus a different atypical antipsychotic

This recommendation is based completely on case studies and reports by expert clinicians

Stage 3A   Lithium plus divalproex or carbamazepine plus alternate atypical antipsychotic

When augmentation treatment (stage 2A) fails the panel recommended substitution of an alternate atypical antipsychotic

Stage 4   Combination of two mood stabilizers plus atypical antipsychotic

When children do not respond to a traditional mood stabilizer and two atypical antipsychotic trails the panel recommended prescribing a combination treatment consisting of two mood stabilizers plus an atypical antipsychotic drug

Lithium plus divalproex or carbamazepine plus an atypical antipsychotic medication is an example of the recommended combination treatment

The recommendation is based only on case studies and clinical reports from experts

Stage 5   Alternate monotherapy plus atypical antipsychotic

If the child fails to respond to any of the treatments recommended in stages 1 to 4 doctors are encouraged to prescribe an alternate monotherapy, such as oxcarbazepine, plus an atypical antipsychotic

The recommendation is based only on case studies and clinical reports from experts

Stage 6   ECT or clozapine

The panel recommended Clozapine for children and adolescents who do not respond when treated with a combination of three medications.

ECT received a recommendation only for adolescents who are medication resistant. Children should not be treated with ECT

The lack of prospective studies prevented the panel from developing an algorithm for treating bipolar I depression in children and adolescents

*Summarized from reference 85

Algorithm for treating childhood manic or mixed episodes complicated with psychosis

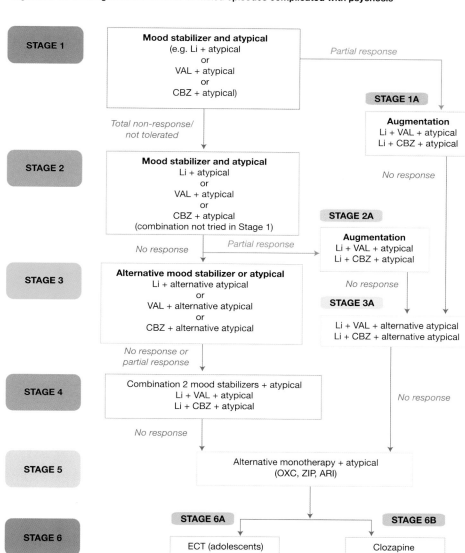

Algorithm 2

Algorithm 3 Algorithm for treating adult depression in bipolar disorder. This algorithm should be utilized in conjunction with the primary treatment algorithm for mania/hypomania. If a patient reports symptoms of depression significant enough to warrant intervention, the clinician is directed to utilize this algorithm as a concomitant treatment strategy, in addition to any stage of treatment within the mania/hypomania algorithm. As with any algorithm, if insufficient response in depressive symptoms is achieved, the clinician should continue through the algorithm until satisfactory symptom reduction is achieved. It is important to consider carefully the addition of an antidepressant to a bipolar patient's medication regimen. If the patient presents with a 'pure' bipolar major depressive episode, without mood lability or hypomania, the decision is relatively clear, as the degree of suffering will justify initiating an antidepressant. However, many patients will have significant depressive symptoms, but also periods of dysphoric hypomania, mood lability, irritability, and other complicated states. Patients may need both a mood stabilizer and an antidepressant. The balancing of optimizing mood stabilizers, possibly adding lithium, or adding an antidepressant, must be done on a case-by-case basis.

The algorithm to treat bipolar depression assumes that antidepressants will only be used in conjunction with a mood-stabilizing medication, because of the risk of inducing manic symptoms. It may be necessary to adjust the mood stabilizer during treatment (i.e. increasing the dose with development of irritability or mood lability). In some cases it may be clinically indicated to switch or combine mood stabilizers (i.e. if an effective antidepressant is found and continued need for the medication is provided, but the drug is associated with mild mood lability). It is expected that the physician will continue to utilize recommendations of the hypomania/mania algorithm even when prescribing antidepressant treatment.

Selection of a specific antidepressant medication should be made based on individual factors such as the expected side-effect profile, potential toxicity, concomitant medical problems, and medications. The initial algorithm stages focus on antidepressant monotherapy with medications associated with favorable risk–benefit ratios and for which there is evidence of efficacy in bipolar patients.

Stage 1   The first stage includes initiating and/or optimizing mood-stabilizing medications. The recommendation is that all patients diagnosed with bipolar I disorder be prescribed antimanic medications, using the algorithm for treatment of mania/hypomania. The committee made explicit the recommendation that optimizing mood-stabilizing medications might mean either an increase or a decrease in dosing, although no data are available to direct tactics clearly on this issue.

Stage 2   Patients entering Stage 2 of the algorithm should have a major depressive episode of sufficient severity to merit medication treatment. Stage 2 includes the addition of a selective serotonin reuptake inhibitor (SSRI), bupropion SR, or lamotrigine to existing medications. The SSRI options are open, and include fluoxetine, paroxetine, sertraline, fluvoxamine, and citalopram. Bupropion SR is an additional option (the committee recommended the sustained-release version of bupropion, due to improved tolerability). While there is a risk of rash with lamotrigine, there are positive Level A data in support of its efficacy for treatment of bipolar depression.

Stage 3   At this point, the algorithm begins to rely more heavily on clinical consensus and expert opinion, as there are only limited data on treatment of bipolar depression following failure in Stage 2. The algorithm development philosophy was that when there are several options available, with little or no empirically derived reason to rank them, choices should be offered so that the clinician and patient can choose what is best for that individual. Therefore, Stage 3 offers the clinician and patient several options, including addition of lithium, switching to an alternative antidepressant medication (adding venlafaxine and nefazodone as additional options), or adding from Stage 2 options a second antidepressant or lamotrigine. If Stage 2 treatment was unsuccessful primarily because of intolerable side-effects, consider selecting an antidepressant from a different class with a contrasting side-effect profile (e.g. if the patient experienced sexual dysfunction on an SSRI, consider bupropion SR or nefazodone).

Stage 4   This stage includes the combination of two antidepressant medications. This includes selection from the SSRI group, bupropion SR, and lamotrigine. In choosing an antidepressant combination, it is recommended to use medications from different classes (i.e. not two SSRIs). The goal of combination antidepressant regimens is to combine medications to enhance clinical response. In general, because of the potential for drug interactions, antidepressant combination treatment should be used carefully, and patients monitored closely.

Stage 5   This stage includes changing the antidepressant medication to an MAOI, or adding an atypical antipsychotic medication. Because of potential health risks and the need to follow special dietary restrictions and avoid certain medications, MAOIs are located in Stage 5, after medications and medication combinations with fewer Level A and B data. Diet-restriction guidelines should be provided to all patients receiving MAOI medications.

Stage 6   Recommendations at this stage include using the alternative not used in Stage 5, ECT, or Other. The 'Other' category is exploratory, and includes a number of options to be considered in addition to partially effective medication combinations. It includes inositol, dopamine agonists, stimulant medications, thyroid, conventional

Algorithm for treating adult bipolar depression

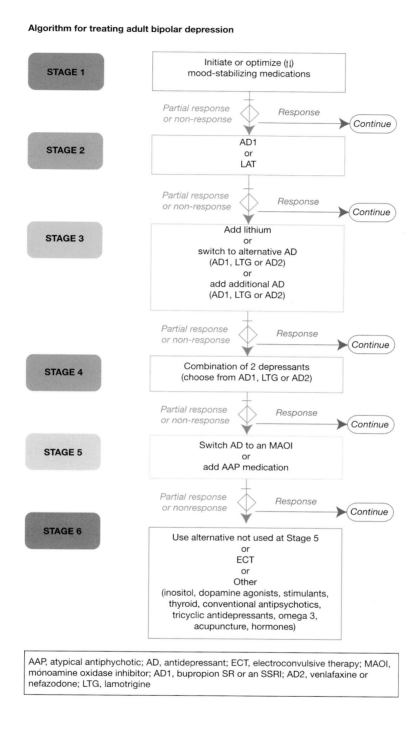

AAP, atypical antiphychotic; AD, antidepressant; ECT, electroconvulsive therapy; MAOI, mónoamine oxidase inhibitor; AD1, bupropion SR or an SSRI; AD2, venlafaxine or nefazodone; LTG, lamotrigine

Algorithm 3

antipsychotics, tricyclic antidepressants, omega 3, acupuncture and hormones. Consultation with the module director, Dr Suppes, is available if a clinician is considering treatment from Stage 7 for a patient who achieved no or partial response to all other algorithm options.

Reproduced with permission from reference 25

Algorithm 4 Algorithm for adult mania/hypomania. This is the primary treatment algorithm. All patients diagnosed with bipolar I disorder should be treated with medication or medication combinations recommended within this guideline. Consistent with other published guidelines for treatment of bipolar disorder, the majority of treatment options consist of medication combinations. If possible, when adjusting medications, it is preferable to make adjustments to one agent at a time, to allow for evaluation of response.

When utilizing mood-stabilizing medications, it is recommended that the dose be pushed (either alone or in combination) as much as possible before moving to the second or third mood stabilizer. Switching to alternative mood stabilizers, versus adding, is recommended in cases of intolerance. If a patient has no or low-partial response to a medication, and is tolerating the medication, a new medication should be added using the overlap and taper tactics provided. It is recommended that the clinician try to taper the first medication at a later date if the patient's mood stabilizes.

When treating patients with hypomania or mania, a first consideration involves decreasing and/or discontinuing antidepressant medications. This taper should be done relatively quickly, except in cases where it is contraindicated. For those patients with rapid cycling, antidepressants should be tapered and discontinued. Some patients may still need an antidepressant plus mood stabilizers in order to minimize depressive symptoms and suicidality.

Serum levels: If lithium or divalproex sodium are utilized, serum levels are part of the consideration of response and tolerability. In practice, serum levels may not be available at each visit. It is recommended that by 2 weeks after initiating lithium or divalproex sodium the patient be receiving the minimum target dose. If possible, we recommend a serum level 5 days after reaching the target dose and before the first appointment to assess response (e.g. 2–3 weeks after starting the trial). While awaiting serum levels (e.g. 4 weeks), it is generally safe to gradually increase divalproex sodium and, more cautiously, lithium if no side-effects develop.

Target serum levels are provided in Table 6.6. For lithium and divalproex sodium evidence supports differences in clinical response for some patients between therapeutic and high therapeutic levels. Clinically, it is reasonably safe and well tolerated to exceed the recommended therapeutic range for divalproex sodium (> 125 µg/ml), but few psychiatric patients appear to need these higher levels. The upper limits of lithium (1.2 mmol/l) are usually associated with side-effects, and levels over these limits are potentially toxic, with the exception of patients in a full-blown manic episode, who may tolerate and benefit from levels of lithium between 1.0 and 1.2 mmol/l.

Similarly, it is necessary to obtain more frequent levels of divalproex sodium when used in combination with an autoinducer such as carbamazepine. Once a couple of levels have been obtained for divalproex sodium or lithium, it is generally possible to estimate the likely increase of serum levels with dose changes and collect serum levels somewhat less often. However, the development of side-effects should always signal considering obtaining a serum level.

Stage 1	All the options for Stage 1 include monotherapy with either lithium, divalproex sodium, or olanzapine. For patients presenting with euphoric mania/hypomania or psychotic mania, choice is from any of the three agents. For dysphoric or mixed mania, the recommendation is to choose between divalproex sodium and olanzapine. Divalproex sodium is recommended instead of valproic acid due to significantly better tolerability. Generally, in the case of partial response with good tolerance, the recommendation will be to add a medication (move to combination therapy, i.e. Stage 2) versus switching. If the patient is intolerant in Stage 1, the recommendation will be to try an alternative mood stabilizer within Stage 1.
Stage 2	In this stage treatment includes combination therapy with two of the following: lithium (Li), divalproex sodium, oxcarbazepine, olanzapine, and risperidone. Oxcarbazepine and risperidone are added as options here. Oxcarbazepine is recommended over carbamazepine due to its apparent similar efficacy with fewer drug interactions and adverse events, increased tolerability, and less physician supervision required. Therefore, the combination is (Li or AC) + AC, or (Li or AC) + AAP, where AC = anticonvulsant and AAP = atypical antipsychotic.
Stage 3	In this stage, physicians are asked to attempt another combination of medications, drawing from the same group described in Stage 2. Preferably, they would keep one agent from the previous combination, and change to a different second agent. Again, the combination can be either (Li or AC) + AC or (Li or AC) + AAP.
Stage 4	This stage also includes combination therapy, but at this point the physician is prompted directly to use an atypical antipsychotic agent in combination with lithium, divalproex, or oxcarbazepine. (Li or AC) + AAP. For patients with psychotic mania, the recommendation is to progress immediately to this combination if Stage 1 monotherapy with either lithium, divalproex sodium, or olanzapine is ineffective or only partially effective. Quetiapine and ziprasidone are added as additional choices here.
Stage 5	This stage includes 'triple therapy,' with lithium, an anticonvulsant (choose from divalproex sodium or oxcarbazepine), and an atypical antipsychotic medication (choose from olanzapine, risperidone, quetiapine, ziprasidone): Li + AC + AAP.

Algorithm for treating adult mania/hypomania

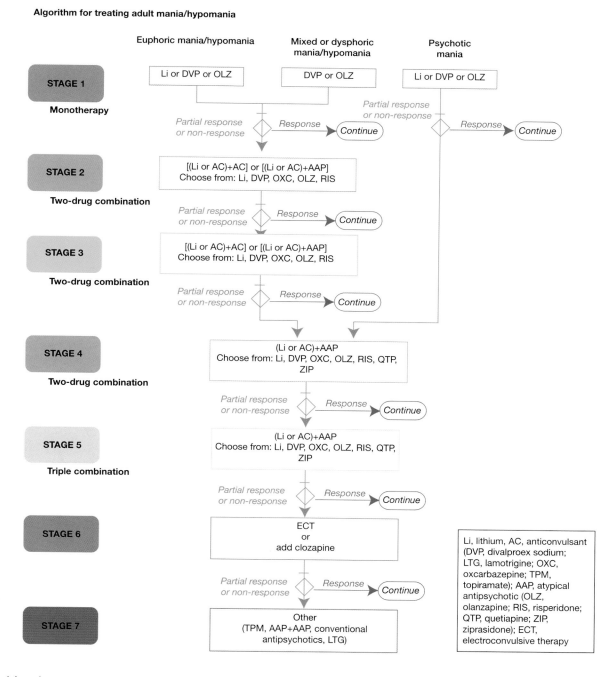

Algorithm 4

Stage 6   ECT has demonstrated efficacy for treatment of acute mania. Safety, tolerability, and patient acceptance issues warrant its placement further down in the algorithm at Stage 6. Alternatively, clozapine could be added to other medications as a treatment option here. The placement of clozapine after other atypical antipsychotic medications is consistent with clinical recommendations to attempt treatment with other atypical antipsychotic medications before initiating clozapine treatment. If the patient is taking clozapine, weekly blood draws (white blood cells) are necessary.

Stage 7   This stage includes other options to be used as adjuncts to partially effective medication combinations. These are topiramate, a combination of medications that includes two atypical antipsychotic medications, conventional antipsychotics, and lamotrigine.

Reproduced with permission from reference 25

PSYCHOTHERAPY FOR BIPOLAR DISORDERS

While medication is the primary intervention for treating bipolar disorders, psychotherapy can help the person and family to cope better with the illness, periods of normalcy between episodes, and the chaotic world caused by mental illness. Patients generally report that both cognitive and interpersonal psychotherapy models provide help and support[17]. However, only supportive therapy is provided until a complete assessment and diagnosis has been completed and the person is introduced to medication. An illustrated review of symptoms that often cluster with bipolar disorder has been provided.

In all models of therapy, one of the most important elements is the relationship between patient and therapist. The therapeutic alliance is strengthened when therapists demonstrate an extensive knowledge of bipolar disorder, an ability to explain basic brain functioning and the role of medication, and honest compassion[1]. Therapist flexibility is a key requirement for managing psychotherapy with individuals who have bipolar disorders. The very nature of the illness forces shifts in treatment focus, changes in emphasis, and the need to redefine goals. As an example, psychoeducation is often focused on as a first step in therapy. However, it may suddenly regain importance when a patient who is doing well starts thinking about stopping the use of medications. Furthermore, during acute episodes, psychotherapy shifts into a concrete supportive and monitoring role. Particularly during periods of severe bipolar depression, patients need trusted reassurance and constant monitoring for signs of suicidal thoughts and behaviors.

To navigate the waters of psychotherapy in patients who have bipolar disorders, this author has for years used a modular eclectic framework for guiding talk therapy. The structure is largely founded on neuroscience theory, and employs behavioral–cognitive methods along with elements of problem-solving, self-understanding, and existential interventions. Before therapy is initiated, clients are assured that bipolar illness is a true brain disorder that cannot be cured by psychotherapy. The role of Modular Eclectic Psychotherapy (MEP) is to help patients cope better with symptoms, remain on medication regimens, improve interpersonal relationships, better understand and accept themselves,

and improve or further develop personal strengths. A central theme in the model is the inclusion of family and significant others in the therapy and in the flow of information. There will be patients who do not want their family to participate, or have no family in the immediate area. Requests not to invite and work with family members must be ethically and legally honored. However, inclusion of family members or significant others within the MEP model is not dropped. Periodically the therapist is expected to explore with the client how and on what terms family members can be invited to participate. Furthermore, with the patient's permission, phone conferences using speaker phones and email can allow distant family members to join selected therapy sessions.

Resistance to family participation is sometimes bridged as the therapeutic relationship grows, and the patient learns that the therapist respects and protects the person's confidentiality and privacy needs. Some patients, however, cannot include their family until a written contract is hammered out, guaranteeing that certain issues and boundaries will be protected. Bipolar disorders disrupt and make interpersonal relationships difficult for the patient and significant others. Therefore, psychotherapy must work toward normalizing, healing, and enhancing long-term family and support systems. To accomplish this, the MEP system incorporates numerous treatment theories and methods into the following 11 modules:

(1) Education;

(2) Symptom monitoring;

(3) General support;

(4) Specific support;

(5) Focused psychotherapy;

(6) Cognitive restructuring and clarification;

(7) Behavior awareness, reinforcement, and modification;

(8) Personal insight and understanding;

(9) Existential psychotherapy;

(10) Termination;

(11) Booster sessions.

This approach has grown out of over 25 years of the author's clinical practice, observations, and conversations with patients and their families. Each of the modules incorporates and borrows from a host of psychotherapy methods and helping skills that have been researched and perfected over the years by countless master therapists. MEP is a framework designed to help the therapist plan a comprehensive therapeutic approach for addressing the multifaceted problems and strengths of people whose lives have been complicated by serious psychiatric illnesses. The efficacy of using psychotherapy as an add-on to medication treatment for patients with bipolar disorders is well documented and accepted[1,17,18]. A list of references supporting the importance, role and effectiveness of, and major methods used in psychotherapy is provided below. However, the following rules, beliefs, values, and concepts capture the philosophy and spirit of the MEP framework:

(1) The therapist must continuously reassess the person for mania, depression, psychosis, substance abuse, suicide, and anxiety.

(2) The order in which the modules and methods are applied depends on the client's needs and the environmental context. The therapist is responsible for transitioning to the most appropriate module as changes occur in the patient's illness, personal and family needs, and environment.

(3) The therapist needs to know more about bipolar disorders, medication, and psychotherapy than the patient.

(4) Psychotherapy stops or shifts to a concrete supportive role during periods of mania, severe depression, or psychosis.

(5) The therapist must always be ready to shift from therapy to support.

(6) The involvement of family and significant others in treatment planning, information sharing, education, support, and problem-solving is a constant treatment goal.

(7) Family members are periodically included in therapy sessions, and an attempt is made always to include family members during periods of crises and when major treatment, life, time, or economic decisions are to be made.

(8) Treatment should never isolate the patient from the family and significant others, and treatment

as often as possible should include the family and significant others.

(9) The perceptions, observations, beliefs, concerns, and culture of the patient and family are not only listened to, but also validated and respected, and, when not in conflict with sound treatment, incorporated into the psychotherapy process. Not all beliefs and cultural perspectives are congruent with best-practice methods. As an example, a belief that depression is a choice cannot go unchallenged or be validated and turned into a treatment method or goal.

(10) Psychotherapy techniques may be presented alone, or in parallel with other strategically planned psychotherapeutic methods.

(11) The patient's treatment compliance and the effectiveness of treatment is reviewed during each session. The therapist, patient, and family must determine whether:

(a) Compliance is helping to stabilize or increase the client's functioning;

(b) Lack of compliance is an indicator of increased symptoms or an indicator of a need for changes in the treatment plan.

(12) Each session surveys not only the patient's and family's problems, but also the successes and strengths experienced during the week.

(13) Assessments for suicide and hazardous behaviors are conducted in each session.

Within the framework's neurosciencific theory, humanistic philosophy, and value system, therapy sessions move purposefully across the 11 modules. The key emphasis of these modules is briefly outlined below. It is beyond the scope of this book to provide or even list all of the elements that can be contained in the independent modules. Nonetheless, the primary purpose of each module is provided. It becomes the therapist, patient, and family's responsibility to develop individualized and meaningful treatment goals within each module and across the framework.

Education module Patients, families, and significant others are helped to understand why bipolar disorders are brain illnesses, the cause of illness, why medication is needed, and rules for taking medications. This module also includes information on methods for coping with symptoms, changing energy levels and motivation, changing personal and family requirements, and how to address work and school problems better. An important part of the module is helping patients and families to accept the illness better and plan how to care for each other more effectively. Within this module therapists may want to use numerous handouts. Questionnaires and medication/illness educational forms are included with this section. The medication and illness illustrations (Algorithms 3 and 4) are reprinted with permission from the Texas Medication Algorithm Project.

Symptom monitoring module The primary purpose of this module is to teach patients and families how to keep records of symptoms and important strengths. Systematically illustrating how symptoms and strengths change can greatly help to improve both medication and psychotherapy interventions. Tracking behaviors provides a concrete picture of the patient's progress or increasing problems. There are numerous published rating scales available for helping patients and therapists to quantify and track how symptoms and strengths change over time. Readers will find a series of questionnaires in Appendix 2 of this book that also serve this purpose. Questionnaires, unlike scales, do not provide a total score. Each question is independent and is not considered in relation to other items. Because of the unique nature and circumstances of severe mental illness, scales often lack true psychometric reliability and validity. The use of questionnaires that do not have summative scores partially overcomes this problem. The main purpose of the questionnaires is to serve as a concrete communication tool between the therapist, patient, and family.

General support module Patients and families need ongoing general support. This module is used to provide case management, advocacy, support, and a concrete focus on the patient's and family's strengths. In order to overcome the stresses caused by illness and everyday life, people need to be reminded that they are important and rewarded concretely and verbally for succeeding. The concrete support may be a simple cup of coffee that was not expected, or a willingness by the therapist to change an appointment or help resolve a clinic-related problem. Therapy for chronic problems is enhanced and more meaningful when general support is consistently provided. Patients and family should not have to wait for a crisis before therapists offer concrete

and verbal support. The patient and family should leave therapy sessions feeling validated, important, and reassured.

Specific support module There are times when every patient and family needs an advocate and specific help. The therapist must be prepared either to provide the required support, or to link the individual and family to an agency or professional person who can resolve the difficulty and stress. In addition, during depressive and manic episodes the therapist:

(1) Helps the patient and family to identify tasks that must be completed;

(2) Jointly develops a plan and means for completing the tasks;

(3) Gives the family and patient 'permission' not to perform or to delay work and daily maintenance tasks that can be delayed;

(4) Reminds the patient and family of strengths and validates skills that continue to function even though the patient's illness is not improving or increasing.

During a crisis or severe episode, it may be more productive to direct the family and patient's focus toward recalling that strengths and skills during past episodes disappeared and returned. That is, to overcome despair, individuals are reminded that past severe episodes have been survived, and lost skills regained. Furthermore, the fact that difficult situations and crises caused by illness have been over and again survived is cognitively reframed and reinforced as a current and admirable strength.

Focused psychotherapy module Modified reality-oriented therapy methods are empathetically applied to help the patient and family cope during periods of hypomanic episodes and dangerous periods of depression. The therapist, as an example, becomes the voice of reality and provides specific directives and suggestions for organizing the family, and establishing needed rules. Directives may include specific instructions such as to remove the patient's car keys or to lock up all items that could easily be used for a suicide attempt. During this period it is helpful to increase therapy and home visits. Home visits are difficult and time-consuming, but can:

(1) Provide the therapist with invaluable assessment information;

(2) Aid in helping families know how to handle difficult situations;

(3) Provide information upon which indicators for hospitalization or emergency room treatment can be developed.

It is sometimes helpful during hypomanic and depressed episodes to remind patients cognitively what 'normal' is like, compared with current manic or depressed thoughts and behavior. This can sometimes be accomplished by reviewing past logs, charts, and questionnaires with the patient. With patients who are not agitated or angry, visits and reports from trusted friends or religious leaders or teachers sometimes helps the person to reconstitute and more willingly accept treatment requirements such as constant supervision or hospitalization. The therapist focuses on making a realistic plan that addresses the severity level and immediate needs of the patient and family. If medications are not working and the illness escalates, focused psychotherapy methods will not be helpful. Patients in the midst of a severe depression or mania often need in-patient hospitalization. Additionally, severe depression or mania may spiral into psychosis. During psychotic periods, psychotherapy provides concrete support and case-management services to the patient and family. However, between episodes, this module may also be used for addressing personal, family, and developmental issues that are not specifically related to illness.

Cognitive restructuring and clarification module An important part of psychotherapy is helping people to understand and know how to cope positively with their symptoms, medication side-effects, and routine problems. It can be extremely helpful, as an example, for patients to be able to identify the difference between their 'natural' highs and lows from the behaviors and moods that signal the onset of depression and mania. Furthermore, cognitive restructuring allows patients to reframe their strengths into meaningful and useful structures and schemata.

Behavior awareness, reinforcement, and modification module Standard reward systems can shape behaviors that increase the patient's social skills and decrease actions that limit their successes and quality of life. While positive reinforcement takes longer to change behaviors, the change will outlast changes achieved by punishment. Families sometimes find this difficult to put into practice, but with guidance they most often meet with success.

Personal insight and understanding module When symptoms are in remission, patients have the opportunity to explore themselves as unique individuals. Many are looking for help and guidance for exploring question such as 'Who am I', 'Why do I act this way', or 'How do my personality, temperament, past experiences, and learning support interact with both my strengths and symptoms?' This can be hazardous if clients are allowed to develop false logic or incorrectly link past developmental and social events for explaining their illness. The focus needs to be firmly anchored in the present.

Existential psychotherapy module Patients and families need to understand that with bipolar disorder a person may have more limited life choices, but nonetheless they often do have choices. As an example, one cannot make a choice to stop being depressed, and even the choice to enter or remain out of the hospital may have disappeared. In situations of this type, the therapist's job is to help the patient discover the choices that remain within the restricted circumstances. It is important to keep in mind, however, that both depression and mania can rob a person even of the choice of attitude. This is why sometimes decisions must be made for the patient. While it is important not to promote helplessness, it is nonetheless also crucial for people with an illness to accept and live within their limitations. Furthermore, it is sometimes therapeutic for patients for a short period of time to stop trying to fight their way out of depression. Existentially, patients may make progress by accepting that they do have depressive episodes, exploring the boundaries of the illness, and learning to live more productively within the boundaries. That is, the patient does not have a choice not to become depressed, but, with help, some patients can find positive choices within the walls of their illness. Additionally, during periods of symptom remission, clients can work on learning to accept having bipolar illness, and explore the question, 'Why me?' Perhaps, however, the most important purpose of this module is helping patients and families to learn to make sense of and derive meaning from their difficult situation. It can be helpful for patients and families to discover how the illness has not only given them heartache, but also taught them important unique lessons, forcing them to become perhaps kinder, stronger, smarter, or more understanding. The purpose is not to downplay the negatives of chronic illness, but rather to help patients and families to examine the flip-side of the hardships.

Termination module Psychotherapy ends for many reasons. Patients move, grow tired of sessions, or currently no longer need the support and cognitive interventions that psychotherapy provides. More than simply saying goodbye, the termination module is used to examine what has and has not been accomplished and make plans for how future episodes and crises can be managed. An important termination task is ensuring that the patient and family know the signs signaling the need for emergency medical help or psychotherapy support.

Booster sessions module Many patients find it helpful to return every 4 months or so for 1–3 psychotherapy sessions. Keeping in mind that bipolar disorders are not cured, booster sessions allow the patient and family to maintain a relationship with the therapist, and share how they are changing. When the patient is not having any specific problems, the booster session offers an opportunity for the patient and therapist to explore and deepen their relationship and knowledge of each other. That is, the session is used for providing general support to the patient and sharing appropriate information that builds empathy and respect between the therapist and patient. Every booster session assesses the patient's progress, medication compliance, symptoms, and strengths. The sessions also provide time to clarify issues and ensure that the patient recalls how to know whether emergency medical help or psychotherapy assistance is needed. If the assessment indicates that the patient has unaddressed problems, a plan for resolving the issues or gaining appropriate help can be developed.

Psychotherapy for patients with bipolar disorders will constantly shift within and between these modules. Clients with a severe illness and multiple episodes occurring close together may never experience all of the modalities. The goal is not to push the patient through all of the modules as if they were stages, but rather to have a flexible framework that quickly adapts to the cognitive, emotional, and interpersonal needs of the patient and family.

REFERENCES

1. Goodwin FK, Jamison KR. Manic–Depressive Illness. New York: Oxford University Press, 1990.

2. Taylor EH. Manic Depression. In Ramachandran VS, ed. Encyclopedia of the Human Brain. San Diego: Academic Press, 2002: 2: 745–57.

3. Bowden CL, Singh VS. Long-term management of bipolar disorder. In Medscape, 2003. http://www.medscape.com/viewprogram/2686.

4. Bentley KJ, Walsh JF. The Social Worker and Psychotropic Medication, 2nd edn. Belmont, CA: Wadsworth/Thompson Learning, 2001.

5. Krishnan KRR. Monoamine oxidase inhibitors. In Schatzberg AF, NEmeroff CB, eds. The American Psychiatric Publishing Textbook of Psychopharmacology, 3rd edn. Washington, DC: American Psychiatric Publishing, 2004: 303–14.

6. Stahl SM. Essential Psychopharmacology Neuroscientific Basis and Practical Applications, 2nd edn. New York: Cambridge University Press, 2003.

7. Bezchlibnyk-Butler KZ, Jeffries JJ, eds. Clinical Handbook of Psychotropic Drugs. Toronto: Hogrefe & Huber, 2003.

8. Francois B, Marquet P, Roustan J, et al. Serotonin syndrome due to an overdose of moclobemide and clomipramine: a potentially life-threatening association. Intens Care Med 1997; 23: 122–4.

9. Hodgman MJ, Martin TG, Krenzelok EP. Serotonin syndrome due to venlafaxine and maintenance tranylcypromine therapy. Hum Exp Toxicol 1997; 16: 14–17.

10. Kolecki P. Venlafaxine induced serotonin syndrome occurring after abstinence from phenelzine for more than two weeks [letter]. J Toxicol Clin Toxicol 1997; 35: 211–12.

11. Marangell LB, Silver JM, Goff DC, Yudofsky SC. Psychopharmacology and electroconvulsive therapy. In Hales RE, Yudofsky SC, eds. The American Psychiatric Publishing Textbook of Clinical Psychiatry, 4th edn. Washington, DC: American Psychiatric Publishing, 2003: 1047–149.

12. Beasley CM, Masica D, Heilgenstein JH, et al. Possible monoamine oxidase inhibitor–serotonin uptake inhibitor interaction: fluoxetine clinical data

and preclinical findings. J Clin Psychopharmacol 1993; 13: 312–20.

13. Garlow SJ, Purselle D, D'Orio B. Psychiatric emergencies. In Schatzberg AF, Nemeroff CB, eds. The American Psychiatric Publishing Textbook of Psychopharmacology, 3rd edn. Washington, DC: American Psychiatric Publishing, 2004: 1067–82.

14. Akriskal HS. Dysthymic and cyclothymic depressions: therapeutic considerations. Compr Psychiatry 1994; 55 (Suppl 4): 46–52.

15. Rosenbaum JF, Fava M, Nierenberg AA, et al. Treatment resistant mood disorders. In Gabbard GO, ed. Treatment of Psychiatric Disorders. Washington, DC: American Psychiatric Press, 1995: 1275–328.

16. Sachs GS, Printz DJ, Kahn DA, et al. The Expert Consensus Guideline Series: Medication Treatment of Bipolar Disorder. Postgrad Med 2000; 108: 1–104.

17. Hirschfeld RMA, Bowden CL, Gitlin MJ, et al. Practice guideline for the treatment of patients with bipolar disorder. In McIntyre JS, Charles SC, eds. American Psychiatric Association Practice Guidelines for the Treatment of Psychiatric Disorders Compendium 2004. Arlington, VA: American Psychiatric Association, 2004: 525–612.

18. Doubovsky SL, Davis R, Dubovsky AN. Mood disorders. In Hales RE, Yudofsky SC, eds. The American Psychiatric Publishing Textbook of Clinical Psychiatry, 4th edn. Washington, DC: American Psychiatric Publishing, 2003: 439–542.

19. Judd LL, Akiskal HS, Schettler PJ, et al. The long-term natural history of the weekly symptomatic status of bipolar I disorder. Arch Gen Psychiatry 2002; 59: 530–7.

20. Hirschfeld RMA, Goodwin G, Herman E, et al. Stabilizing Depression in Bipolar Disorder. New York: Postgraduate Institute for Medicine, 2004 (http://www.medscape.com/viewprogram/2966_pnt).

21. Post RM, Denicoff KD, Levenrich GS. Presentations of depression in bipolar illness. Clin Neurosci Res 2002; 2: 142–57.

22. Sachs GS, Lafer B, Truman CJ, et al. Lithium monotherapy: miracle, myth and misunderstanding. Psychiatr Ann 1994; 24: 299–306.

23. Zornberg GL, Pope HG. Treatment of depression in bipolar disorder: new directions for research. J Clin Psychopharmacol 1993; 13: 397–408.

24. Grunze H, Kasper S, Goodwin G, et al. The World Federation of Societies of Biological Psychiatry guidelines for biological treatment of bipolar disorders, part I: Treatment of bipolar depression. World J Biol Psychiatry 2002; 3: 115–24.

25. Suppes T, Dennehy EB. Bipolar Disorder Algorithms Manual, Texas Medication Algorithm Project. Austin, TX: Department of Mental Health and Mental Retardation; Dallas, TX: University of Texas Southwestern Medical School, 2002, 2002 (http://www.dshs.state.ex.us/mhprograms/disclaimer.shtm).

26. Bhagwagar Z, Goodwin GM. The role of lithium in the treatment of bipolar depression. Clin Neurosci Res 2002; 2: 222–7.

27. Mondimore FM. Bipolar Disorder: A Guide for Patients and Families. John Hopkins Health Book. Baltimore, MD: Johns Hopkins University Press, 1999.

28. Miklowitz DJ. The Bipolar Disorder Survival Guide: What You and Your Family Need to Know. New York: Guilford Press, 2002.

29. Schatzberg AF, Nemeroff CB, eds. The American Psychiatric Publishing Textbook of Psychopharmacology, 3rd edn. Washington, DC: American Psychiatric Publishing, 2004.

30. Baalstrup P, Schou M. Lithium as a prophylactic agent: its effect against recurrent depressions and manic–depressive psychosis. Arch Gen Psychiatry 1967; 2: 162–72.

31. Zornberg GL, Rose HG. Treatment of depression in bipolar disorder: new directions for research. J Clin Psychopharmacol 1993; 13: 397–408.

32. Goodwin FK, Murphy DL, Bunney WE Jr. Lithium carbonate treatment in depression and mania. Arch Gen Psychiatry 1969; 21: 486–96.

33. Goodwin FK, Murphy DL, Dunner DL, et al. Lithium response in unipolar versus bipolar depression. Am J Psychiatry 1972; 129: 44–7.

34. Goodwin FK, Bowden CL, Calabrese JR, et al. Maintenance treatments for bipolar I depression. In American Psychiatric Association Annual Meeting, May 2003, San Francisco.

35. Bowden CL, Calabrese JR, Sachs GS, et al. A placebo-controlled 18-month trail of lamotrigine and lithium maintenance treatment in recently manic or hypomanic patients with bipolar I disorder. Arch Gen Psychiatry 2003; 60: 392–400.

36. Calabrese JR, Bowden CL, Rheimherr F, et al. Lamotrigine or lithium in the maintenance treatment of bipolar I disorder. In American Psychiatric Association Annual Meeting, May 2002, Philadeplphia, PA.

37. Calabrese J, Bowden CL, Sachs GS, et al. A placebo-controlled 18-month trial of lamotrigine and lithium maintenance treatment in recently depressed patients with bipolar disorder. J Clin Psychiatry 2003; 64: 1013–24.

38. Calabrese JR, Bowden CL. A double-blind placebo-controlled study of lamotrigine monotherapy in outpatients with bipolar I depression. J Clin Psychiatry 1999; 60: 79–88.

39. Herman E, Hovorka J, Syrovatka J, et al. Relapse prevention with lamotrigine in bipolar II disorder. Presented at the 12th World Congress of Psychiatry, Yokohama, Japan, August 2002.

40. Calabrese JR, Vieta E, Shelton MD. Latest maintenance data on lamotrigine in bipolar disorder. Eur Neuropsychopharmacol 2003; 13 (Suppl 2): S57–66.

41. Keck PE, McElroy SL, Strakowski SM, et al. Compliance with maintenance treatment in bipolar disorder. Psychopharmacol Bull 1997; 33: 87–91.

42. Asnis G, Bowden CL, Calabrese JR. Safety and tolerability of lamotrigine in bipolar I disorder. Presented at the 43rd Annual Meeting of the New Clinical Drug Evaluation Unit, Boca Raton, FL May 2003.

43. Martinez-Aran A, Vieta E, Colom F. Cognitive function across manic or hypomanic, depressed, and euthymic states in bipolar disorder. Am J Psychiatry 2004; 161: 262–70.

44. Pachet A, Wisniewski A. The effects of lithium on cognition: an update review. Psychopharmacology 2003; 170: 225–34.

45. Calabrese JR, Sullivan JR, Bowden CL, et al. Rash in multicenter trials of lamotrigine in mood disorders: clinical relevance and management. J Clin Psychiatry 2002; 63: 1012–19.

46. Passmore MJ, Garnham J, Duffy A, et al. Phenotypic spectra of bipolar disorder in response to lithium versus lamotrigine. Bipolar Disord 2003; 5: 110–14.

47. Swann AC, Bowden CL, Calabrese JR, et al. Pattern of response to divalproex, lithium, or placebo in four naturalistic subtypes of mania. Neuropsychopharmacology 2002; 26: 530–6.

48. Peet M, Peter S. Drug-induced mania. Drug Saf 1995; 12: 146–53.

49. Boerlin J, Gitlin MJ, Zoellner LA, et al. Bipolar depression and antidepressant-induced mania: a naturalistic study. J Clin Psychiatry 1998; 59: 374–9.

50. Bottlender R, Rudolf D, Strauss A, et al. Mood-stabilisers reduce the risk for developing antidepressant-induced maniform states in acute treatment of bipolar I depressed patients. J Affect Disord 1998; 63: 79–83.

51. Henry C, Sorbara F, Lacoste J, et al. Antidepressant-induced mania in bipolar patients: identification of risk factors. J Clin Psychiatry 2001; 62: 249–55.

52. Preda A, MacLean RW, Mazure CM, et al. Antidepressant-associated mania and psychosis in psychiatric admissions. J Clin Psychiatry 2001; 62: 30–3.

53. Altshuler L, Trisha S, David B, et al. Impact of antidepressant discontinuation after acute bipolar depression remission on rates of depressive relapse at 1-year follow-up. Am J Psychiatry 2003; 160: 1252–62.

54. Mallakh RS, Karippot A. Use of antidepressants to treat depression in bipolar disorder. Psychiatr Serv 2002; 53: 580–4.

55. Keck PE, Ice KN. Ziprasidone Study Group: controlled treatment of acute mania with ziprasidone. Presented at the American Psychiatric Association 153rd Annual Meeting, Chicago, IL, May 2000.

56. McElroy SL, Keck PE Jr. Pharmacological agents for the treatment of acute bipolar mania. Biol Psychiatry 2000; 48: 539–57.

57. Keck PE Jr, McElroy SL. Treatment of bipolar disorder. In Schatzberg AF, Nemeroff CB, eds. The American Psychiatric Publishing Textbook of Psychopharmacology, 3rd edn. Washington, DC: American Psychiatric Publishing, 2004: 865–84.

58. West SA, Keck PE Jr, McElroy SL. Valproate. In Goodnick PJ, ed. Mania. Washington, DC: American Psychiatric Press, 1998: 301–18.

59. Pope HG, McElroy SL, Keck PE Jr, et al. Valproate in the treatment of acute mania: a placebo-controlled study. Arch Gen Psychiatry 1991; 48: 62–8.

60. Swann AC, Bowden CL, Calabrese JR, et al. Differential effect of number of previous episodes of affective disorder on response to lithium or divalproex in acute mania. Am J Psychiatry 1999; 156: 1264–6.

61. Solomon DA, Ryan CE, Keitner GI, et al. A pilot study of lithium carbonate plus divalproex sodium for the continuation and maintenance treatment of patients with bipolar I disorder. J Clin Psychiatry 1997; 58: 95–9.

62. McElroy SL, Keck PE Jr, Stanton SP, et al. A randomized comparison of divalproex oral loading versus haloperidol in initial treatment of acute psychotic mania. J Clin Psychiatry 1996; 57: 142–6.

63. Tohen M, Baker RW, Altshuler LL, et al. Olanzapine versus valproex in the treatment of acute mania. Am J Psychiatry 2002; 159: 1011–17.

64. Zajecka JM, Weisler R, Swann AC. Divalproex sodium versus olanzapine for the treatment of acute mania in bipolar disorder. In American College of Neuropsychopharmacology Annual Meeting Poster Abstracts, December 2000, Nashville, TN.

65. Namjoshi M, Rajamannar G, Risser R, et al. Impact of olanzapine added to lithium or valproate on the quality of life of patients with bipolar disorder. In Program and Abstracts of the European College of Neuropsychopharmacology, September 2000, Munich.

66. Tohen M, Vieta E, Calabrese J, et al. Efficacy of olanzapine and olanzapine-fluoxetine combination in the treatment of bipolar I depression. Arch Gen Psychiatry 2003, 60:1079-1088.

67. Tohen M, Jacobs TG, Grundy SL, et al. Efficacy of olanzapine in acute bipolar mania: a double-blind, placebo-controlled study. The Olanzapine HGGW Study Group. Arch Gen Psychiatry 2000; 57: 841–9.

68. Tohen M, Sanger TM, McElroy SL, et al. Olanzapine versus placebo in the treatment of acute mania. Am J Psychiatry 1999; 156: 702–9.

69. Yatham LN. Acute and maintenance treatment of bipolar mania: the role of atypical antipsychotics. Bipolar Disord 2003; 5 (Suppl 2): 7–19.

70. Esparon J, Kolloori J, Naylor G, et al. Comparison of the prophylactic action of flupenthixol with placebo in lithium treated manic–depressive patients. Br J Psychiatry 1986; 148: 723–5.

71. Kane J. Tardive dyskinesia in affective disorder. J Clin Psychiatry 1999; 60: 43–7.

72. Shi L, Namjoshi M, Tohen M, et al. Olanzapine versus haloperidol: a prospective comparison of clinical and humanistic outcomes in bipolar disorder. Presented at the 154th Annual American Psychiatric Association Meeting, New Orleans, LA, May 2001: abstr.

73. Torrey EF, Knable MB. Surviving Manic Depression: A Manual on Bipolar Disorder for Patients, Families and Providers. New York: Basic Books, 2002.

74. Regier DA, Farmer ME, Rae DS, et al. Comorbidity of mental disorder with alcohol and other drug abuse: results from the Epidemiologic Catchment Area (ECA) study. JAMA 1990; 264: 2511–18.

75. Regier DA, Boyd JH, Burke JD, et al. One-month prevalence of mental disorders in the United States: based on five Epidemiologic Catchment Area sites. Arch Gen Psychiatry 1988; 45: 977–86.

76. Mueser KT, Noordsy DL, Drake RE, Fox L. Integrated Treatment For Dual Disorders: A Guide to Effective Practice. New York: Guilford Press, 2003.

77. Dorus W, Ostrow DG, Anton R, et al. Lithium treatment of depressed and nondepressed alcoholics. JAMA 1989; 262: 1646–52.

78. Clark DC, Fawcett J. Does lithium carbonate therapy for alcoholism deter relapse drinking? In Galanter M, ed. Recent Developments in Alcoholism, Vol 7. Treatment Research. New York: Plenum Press, 1989: 315–28.

79. de la Fuente JR, Morse RM, Niven RG, et al. A controlled study of lithium carbonate in the treatment of alcoholism. Mayo Clin Proc 1989: 177–80.

80. Wagner KD. Treatment of Childhood and Adolescent Disorders. In Schatzberg AF, Nemeroff CB, eds. The American Psychiatric Publishing Textbook of Psychopharmacology, 3rd edn. Washington, DC: American Psychiatric Publishing, 2004: 949–1002.

81. Geller B, Cooper TB, Sun K, et al. Double blind and placebo controlled study of lithium for adolescent bipolar disorders with secondary substance dependency. J Am Acad Child Adolesc Psychiatry 1998; 37: 171–8.

82. Stober M, Schmidt-Lackner S, Freeman R, et al. Recovery and relapse in adolescents with bipolar affective illnesses: a five-year naturalistic, prospective follow-up. J Am Acad Child Adolesc Psychiatry 1995; 34: 724–31.

83. Finding RL, Garcious BL, McNamara NK, et al. Combination lithium and divalproex sodium treatment of pediatric bipolar disorder. Presented at the 155th Annual Meeting of the American Psychiatric Association, Philadelphia, PA, May 2002: poster.

84. Wilens TE. Straight Talk About Psychiatric Medications for Kids. New York: Guilford Press, 2004.

85. Kowatch RA, Fristad M, Birmaher B, et al. The Child Psychiatric Workgroup on Bipolar Disorder. Treatment guidelines for children and adolescents with bipolar disorder. J Am Acad Child Adolesc Psychiatry, 2005, 44: 213–35.

Conclusion:
Much to Do, Much to Make Us Hopeful

Great strides have been made in understanding bipolar disorders. Yet there is much left to accomplish. Diagnosis across the life span needs to be more accurate and based on less global, overlapping indicators. Currently, mild symptoms blend with acceptable social behaviors and make early detection of bipolar illness difficult if not impossible. Therefore, identification of the illness for most people does not occur until the symptoms slide into a complete and severe episode. Along with improvements in diagnosis, research must also discover risk factors and developmental indicators that have a higher probability of predicting illness onset. Our knowledge of risk factors is so general that developing an aggressive public health prevention program is impossible. This is due in part to research limitations, funding, and the lack of forward-looking public health policies.

The United States has no national registry that allows following the lifetime course of an illness. Furthermore, in the United States, the lack of national health insurance and inequities in the coverage of mental disorders by private insurers prevent many people from being seen by mental health experts when symptoms are mild and a diagnosis is uncertain. Clinics are prohibited from offering services and attempting to prevent bipolar episodes when financial reimbursement requires a DSM or other form of diagnosis. Policy-makers, insurance providers, researchers, and consumers also need to insist on greater accuracy in how mental health assessment reports, treatment plans, and treatment notes are recorded. Global or general records provide almost no help for researchers and can cause incorrect findings. General or careless psychiatric notes

can also penalize and misrepresent patients when they move from one clinic to another.

Patients and families do, however, have reason for hope. Within the major research and treatment communities worldwide, bipolar illnesses are accepted as neurobiological disorders. Furthermore, it is common knowledge that people with this illness require a lifetime of specific medical, environmental, and supportive interventions. As a result, increased importance has been placed on working with a patient's family and the communities where the person resides. There is also reason to believe that the accuracy of methods for diagnosing bipolar disorders will improve greatly. The advancement of SPECT and other scanning techniques illustrates that we are on the edge of discovering neurological markers for diagnosing bipolar disorders. Biological measurements will eventually make diagnoses less dependent on behavioral observations of symptoms.

Future medications and genetic treatments hold the possibility of completely curing or at least controlling bipolar disorders for longer periods of time and with fewer side-effects. Major treatment breakthroughs can be expected as science continues unraveling DNA and the interacting genes responsible for bipolar disorders are discovered. Additionally, stem cell research may also usher in new hope for prevention and treatment. Public policies, laws, and community support systems are slowly, but nonetheless positively, changing. Government mental health planning departments are becoming aware that bipolar disorders attack children, adolescents, adults, and the aged. There is growing interest in studying and improving treatment across the life span. Furthermore, the use of evidence-based or best-

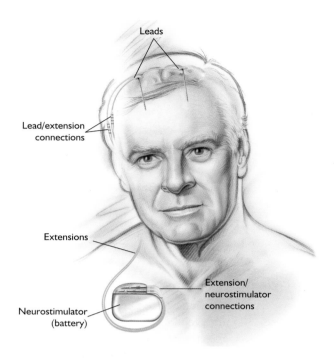

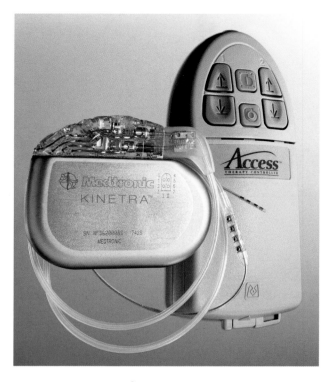

Is this the future for treating unremitting bipolar depression and mania? Science is currently studying the feasibility of using brain pacing technology for treating unipolar depression. As illustrated above the neurostimulator is surgically implanted and delivers electrical stimulation to specific areas located in the brain's right and left hemispheres. The device is similar to pacemakers used for treating heart patients. The treatment process has become known as 'deep brain stimulation'. Medtronic, Inc. and other research oriented companies are studying the effectiveness of the instrument for treating epilepsy, depression, advanced Parkinson's disease and dystonia. Illustration courtesy of Medtronic, Inc. 2005

Medtronic's Kinetra® Dual-Channel Neurostimulator and leads. The devise pictured above has successfully been used in a study of six treatment-resistant patients suffering with unipolar depression. Immediate improvement was experienced by the participating patients. Only a few volts is required for the deep brain stimulation. After six months of treatment four of the six patients continued to have a significant decrease in their depression. Helen Mayberg[1] reported that three patients had almost a complete remission of symptoms. Additionally, none of the participants suffered cognitive or other psychological side effects from the intervention. The electrodes were implanted in the subgenual cingulated region of the brain. The instrument has not been studied with bipolar patients, but may offer hope in the future for individuals with treatment-resistant bipolar depression or mania. Photo courtesy of Medtronic, Inc. 2005

practice methods are starting to be mandated and studied for effectiveness by government agencies. We live in a time of exploding knowledge, and growing scientific awareness. There is solid reason to hope that treatment effectiveness will improve greatly, and social stigma will largely disappear within the lifetime of many who currently have bipolar illness.

REFERENCE

1. Mayberg HS, Lozano AM, Voon V, et al. Deep brain stimulation for treatment resistant depression. Neuron 2005; 45: 651–60.

Appendix 1: Postpartum Questionnaires

INSTRUCTIONS

Clinicians and patients are encouraged jointly to select the questionnaires that parallel either symptoms or issues that need to be tracked. Patients are asked weekly to rate how they perceive each question's level of severity. A unique feature of the questionnaires is that they allow patients to compare their functioning either with illness severity statements or with their capacity when symptoms are in remission. The form's yellow center represents 'normal' functioning. Above the yellow line patients rate identified symptoms and problems. Below the yellow line personal strengths and normal functioning are rated. This provides an opportunity for the patient and clinician to define and identify symptoms, strengths, and periods of normal functioning. These statements can then guide how the patient selects a daily level of functioning.

Feeling depressed or sad: compared to a week without depression how was your mood?							
Week 3	Week 6	Week 9	Week 12	Date____	Date____	Date____	
							A lot: the worst or most difficult possible
							Some: difficult
							A little: somewhat difficult
Baseline: no depression: usual or **normal**. Below categories are used if **overall mood** is normal or better than normal							
							Same or somewhat better than 'normal'
							Much better than 'normal'
							Better than ever experienced
Copyright © 2005 Edward H. Taylor							

Problems completing **daily child-care** tasks							
Week 3	Week 6	Week 9	Week 12	Date____	Date____	Date____	
							A lot: the worst or most difficult possible
							Some: difficult
							A little not done: somewhat difficult
Baseline: no depression: usual or **normal**. Below categories are used only if **daily child-care tasks** are normal or better than normal							
							Same or somewhat better than 'normal'
							Much better than 'normal'
							Better than ever experienced
Copyright © 2005 Edward H. Taylor							

Difficulty **being with** or around the child/children							
Week 3	Week 6	Week 9	Week 12	Date____	Date____	Date____	
							A lot: the worst or most difficult possible
							Some: difficult
							A little: somewhat difficult
Baseline: no depression: usual or **normal**. Below categories are used if **being with child presents no problem**							
							Same or somewhat better than 'normal'
							Much better than 'normal'
							Better than ever experienced
Copyright © 2005 Edward H. Taylor							

Problems in **knowing what to do as a parent**							
Week 3	Week 6	Week 9	Week 12	Date____	Date____	Date____	
							A lot: the worst or most difficult possible
							Some: difficult
							A little: somewhat difficult
Baseline: no depression: usual or **normal**. Below categories are used if **knowing what to do as a parent** is normal or better than normal							
							Same or somewhat better than 'normal'
							Much better than 'normal'
							Better than ever experienced
Copyright © 2005 Edward H. Taylor							

Problems managing feelings of **anger** or **upset with the child/children**							
Week 3	Week 6	Week 9	Week 12	Date____	Date____	Date____	
							A lot: the worst or most difficult possible
							Some: difficult
							A little: somewhat difficult
Baseline: no depression: usual or **normal**. Below categories are used if **anger** or level of feeling **upset** with children is normal or better than normal							
							Same or somewhat better than 'normal'
							Much better than 'normal'
							Better than ever experienced
Copyright © 2005 Edward H. Taylor							

Thoughts that you cannot care for child/children

Week 3	Week 6	Week 9	Week 12	Date____	Date____	Date____	
							A lot: the worst or most difficult possible
							Some: difficult
							A little: somewhat difficult
Baseline: no depression: usual or **normal**. Below categories are used if thoughts about ability to care for child are normal or better than normal							
							Same or somewhat better than 'normal'
							Much better than 'normal'
							Better than ever experienced

Copyright © 2005 Edward H. Taylor

Problems enjoying or having interest in **pleasurable activities**

Week 3	Week 6	Week 9	Week 12	Date____	Date____	Date____	
							A lot: the worst or most difficult possible
							Some: difficult
							A little: somewhat difficult
Baseline: no depression: usual or **normal**. Below categories are used if interest in pleasurable activities is normal or better than normal							
							Same or somewhat better than 'normal'
							Much better than 'normal'
							Better than ever experienced

Copyright © 2005 Edward H. Taylor

Problems with **diet, eating, and weight management**							
Week 3	Week 6	Week 9	Week 12	Date____	Date____	Date____	
							A lot: the worst or most difficult possible
							Some: difficult
							A little: somewhat difficult
Baseline: no depression: usual or **normal**. Below categories are used if **diet** is normal or better than normal							
							Same or somewhat better than 'normal'
							Much better than 'normal'
							Better than ever experienced

Copyright © 2005 Edward H. Taylor

Problems **sleeping** (includes being awake but unable to get out of bed)							
Week 3	Week 6	Week 9	Week 12	Date____	Date____	Date____	
							A lot: the worst or most difficult possible
							Some: difficult
							A little: somewhat difficult
Baseline: no depression: usual or **normal**. Below categories are used if **sleeping** is normal (not depressed) or better than normal							
							Same or somewhat better than 'normal'
							Much better than 'normal'
							Better than ever experienced

Copyright © 2005 Edward H. Taylor

Fear that you are going to **injure, hurt, or kill** the child/children

Week 3	Week 6	Week 9	Week 12	Date____	Date____	Date____	
							A lot: the worst or most difficult possible
							Some: difficult
							A little: somewhat difficult

Baseline: no depression: usual or **normal**. Below categories are used if you have no problems with **fear of injuring, hurting, or killing** your child/children

							Same or somewhat better than 'normal'
							Much better than 'normal'
							Better than ever experienced

Copyright © 2005 Edward H. Taylor

Worry that something **bad is going to happen** to child/children

Week 3	Week 6	Week 9	Week 12	Date____	Date____	Date____	
							A lot: the worst or most difficult possible
							Some: difficult
							A little: somewhat difficult

Baseline: no depression: usual or **normal**. Below categories are used if **worry about bad things happening to child** is not a problem

							Same or somewhat better than 'normal'
							Much better than 'normal'
							Better than ever experienced

Copyright © 2005 Edward H. Taylor

Problems **giving positive attention** to child/children

Week 3	Week 6	Week 9	Week 12	Date____	Date____	Date____	
							A lot: the worst or most difficult possible
							Some: difficult
							A little: somewhat difficult

Baseline: no depression: usual or **normal**. Below categories are used if overall **ability to give positive attention** is normal or better than normal

							Same or somewhat better than 'normal'
							Much better than 'normal'
							Better than ever experienced

Feeling **overly tired** most of the time

Week 3	Week 6	Week 9	Week 12	Date____	Date____	Date____	
							A lot: the worst or most difficult possible
							Some: difficult
							A little: somewhat difficult

Baseline: no depression: usual or **normal**. Below categories are used if **feeling tired** is normal or better than normal

							Same or somewhat better than 'normal'
							Much better than 'normal'
							Better than ever experienced

Feeling of **hopelessness** or feeling **empty**							
Week 3	Week 6	Week 9	Week 12	Date____	Date____	Date____	
							A lot: the worst or most difficult possible
							Some: difficult
							A little: somewhat difficult
Baseline: no depression: usual or **normal**. Below categories are used if belief or feeling of **hopelessness** or feeling **empty** is normal or better than normal							
							Same or somewhat better than 'normal'
							Much better than 'normal'
							Better than ever experienced
Copyright © 2005 Edward H. Taylor							

Overall **care given to baby/children**							
Week 3	Week 6	Week 9	Week 12	Date____	Date____	Date____	
							Little care given: the worst or most difficult possible
							Half of needed care given or difficult
							Most but not all care given: somewhat difficult
Baseline: no depression: usual or **normal**. Below categories are used if **actual attention and care given to baby/child** is normal or better than normal							
							Same or somewhat better than 'normal'
							Much better than 'normal'
							Better than ever experienced
Copyright © 2005 Edward H. Taylor							

Discomfort from medications: negative physical, emotional, or cognitive reactions caused by medications							
Week 3	Week 6	Week 9	Week 12	Date____	Date____	Date____	
							The worst or most difficult possible
							Difficult
							Somewhat difficult
							Minor difficulty
							No negative reactions
Copyright © 2005 Edward H. Taylor							

Note: call MD or clinical worker if reaction is in the pink (difficult) or red (worst or most difficult) for more than 3 weeks

Appendix 2: Patient Questionnaires

INSTRUCTIONS

Clinicians and patients are encouraged jointly to select the questionnaires that parallel either symptoms or issues that need to be tracked. Patients are asked daily to rate how they perceive each question's level of severity. A unique feature of the questionnaires is that they allow patients to compare their functioning either with illness severity statements or with their capacity when symptoms are in remission. The yellow center of the form represents the area of 'normal' functioning. This provides an opportunity for the patient and clinician to define what normal functioning means for this individual. These statements can then guide how the patient selects a daily level of functioning.

Overall **mood**: compared with a non-depressed day, how was your mood?							
Day 1	Day 2	Day 3	Day 4	Day 5	Day 6	Day 7	
							The worst or most difficult possible
							Difficult
							Somewhat difficult
Baseline: no depression: usual or **normal**. Below categories are used if **functioning or mood** is normal (not depressed) or better than normal							
							Same or somewhat better than 'normal'
							Much better than 'normal'
							Better than ever experienced
Copyright © 2005 Edward H. Taylor							

Overall problems completing required **daily work** (emploment/school) tasks							
Day 1	Day 2	Day 3	Day 4	Day 5	Day 6	Day 7	
							The worst or most difficult possible
							Difficult
							Somewhat difficult
Baseline: no depression: usual or **normal**. Below categories are used if **functioning or mood** is normal (not depressed) or better than normal							
							Same or somewhat better than 'normal'
							Much better than 'normal'
							Better than ever experienced

Copyright © 2005 Edward H. Taylor

Overall problems in **parenting** and/or **family life**							
Day 1	Day 2	Day 3	Day 4	Day 5	Day 6	Day 7	
							The worst or most difficult possible
							Difficult
							Somewhat difficult
Baseline: no depression: usual or **normal**. Below categories are used if **functioning or mood** is normal (not depressed) or better than normal							
							Same or somewhat better than 'normal'
							Much better than 'normal'
							Better than ever experienced

Copyright © 2005 Edward H. Taylor

Overall problems in **decision-making** or **knowing what to do**							
Day 1	Day 2	Day 3	Day 4	Day 5	Day 6	Day 7	
							The worst or most difficult possible
							Difficult
							Somewhat difficult
Baseline: no depression: usual or **normal**. Below categories are used if **functioning or mood** is normal (not depressed) or better than normal							
							Same or somewhat better than 'normal'
							Much better than 'normal'
							Better than ever experienced

Copyright © 2005 Edward H. Taylor

Overall problems managing **anger** or not feeling **upset** with people							
Day 1	Day 2	Day 3	Day 4	Day 5	Day 6	Day 7	
							The worst or most difficult possible
							Difficult
							Somewhat difficult
Baseline: no depression: usual or **normal**. Below categories are used if **functioning or mood** is normal (not depressed) or better than normal							
							Same or somewhat better than 'normal'
							Much better than 'normal'
							Better than ever experienced

Copyright © 2005 Edward H. Taylor

Overall ability to control reoccurring or repetitive **thoughts**							
Day 1	Day 2	Day 3	Day 4	Day 5	Day 6	Day 7	
							The worst or most difficult possible
							Difficult
							Somewhat difficult
Baseline: no depression: usual or **normal**. Below categories are used if **functioning or mood** is normal (not depressed) or better than normal							
							Same or somewhat better than 'normal'
							Much better than 'normal'
							Better than ever experienced

Overall enjoyment or interest in **pleasurable activities**							
Day 1	Day 2	Day 3	Day 4	Day 5	Day 6	Day 7	
							The worst or most difficult possible
							Difficult
							Somewhat difficult
Baseline: no depression: usual or **normal**. Below categories are used if **functioning or mood** is normal (not depressed) or better than normal							
							Same or somewhat better than 'normal'
							Much better than 'normal'
							Better than ever experienced

Overall **diet**, eating, and weight management							
Day 1	Day 2	Day 3	Day 4	Day 5	Day 6	Day 7	
							The worst or most difficult possible
							Difficult
							Somewhat difficult
Baseline: no depression: usual or **normal**. Below categories are used if **functioning or mood** is normal (not depressed) or better than normal							
							Same or somewhat better than 'normal'
							Much better than 'normal'
							Better than ever experienced
Copyright © 2005 Edward H. Taylor							

Overall **sleeping** (includes being awake but unable to get out of bed)							
Day 1	Day 2	Day 3	Day 4	Day 5	Day 6	Day 7	
							The worst or most difficult possible
							Difficult
							Somewhat difficult
Baseline: no depression: usual or **normal**. Below categories are used if **functioning or mood** is normal (not depressed) or better than normal							
							Same or somewhat better than 'normal'
							Much better than 'normal'
							Better than ever experienced
Copyright © 2005 Edward H. Taylor							

Overall problems in **thinking** or **memory**

Day 1	Day 2	Day 3	Day 4	Day 5	Day 6	Day 7	
							The worst or most difficult possible
							Difficult
							Somewhat difficult

Baseline: no depression: usual or **normal**. Below categories are used if **functioning or mood** is normal (not depressed) or better than normal

							Same or somewhat better than 'normal'
							Much better than 'normal'
							Better than ever experienced

Copyright © 2005 Edward H. Taylor

Overall problems **managing anger** or not feeling **upset** with people

Day 1	Day 2	Day 3	Day 4	Day 5	Day 6	Day 7	
							The worst or most difficult possible
							Difficult
							Somewhat difficult

Baseline: no depression: usual or **normal**. Below categories are used if **functioning or mood** is normal (not depressed) or better than normal

							Same or somewhat better than 'normal'
							Much better than 'normal'
							Better than ever experienced

Copyright © 2005 Edward H. Taylor

Overall feeling of **depression**							
Day 1	Day 2	Day 3	Day 4	Day 5	Day 6	Day 7	
							The worst or most difficult possible
							Difficult
							Somewhat difficult
Baseline: no depression: usual or **normal**. Below categories are used if **functioning or mood** is normal (not depressed) or better than normal							
							Same or somewhat better than 'normal'
							Much better than 'normal'
							Better than ever experienced
Copyright © 2005 Edward H. Taylor							

Discomfort from medications: negative physical, emotional, or cognitive reactions caused by medications							
Day 1	Day 2	Day 3	Day 4	Day 5	Day 6	Day 7	
							The worst or most difficult possible
							Difficult
							Somewhat difficult
							Minor difficulty
							No negative reactions
Copyright © 2005 Edward H. Taylor							

Note: call MD or clinical worker if reaction is in the pink (difficult) or red (worst or most difficult) for more than 3 weeks

Index